Enhancing the Quality of Care in the ICU

Editor

ROBERT C. HYZY

CRITICAL CARE CLINICS

www.criticalcare.theclinics.com

Consulting Editor
RICHARD W. CARLSON

January 2013 • Volume 29 • Number 1

ELSEVIER

1600 John F. Kennedy Blvd., • Suite 1800 • Philadelphia, Pennsylvania 19103-2899

http://www.theclinics.com

CRITICAL CARE CLINICS Volume 29, Number 1
January 2013 ISSN 0749-0704, ISBN-13: 978-1-4557-7075-5

Editor: Patrick Manley
Developmental Editor: Donald Mumford

Critical Care Clinics (ISSN: 0749-0704) is published quarterly by Elsevier Inc., 360 Park Avenue South, New York, NY 10010-1710. Months of issue are January, April, July, and October. Business and Editorial Offices: 1600 John F. Kennedy Blvd., Suite 1800, Philadelphia, PA 19103-2899. Customer Service Office: 6277 Sea Harbor Drive, Orlando, FL 32887-4800. Periodicals postage paid at New York, NY and additional mailing offices. Subscription prices are $193.00 per year for US individuals, $463.00 per year for US institution, $94.00 per year for US students and residents, $238.00 per year for Canadian individuals, $574.00 per year for Canadian institutions, $278.00 per year for international individuals, $574.00 per year for international institutions and $137.00 per year for Canadian and foreign students/residents. To receive student/resident rate, orders must be accompanied by name of affiliated institution, date of term, and the signature of program/residency coordinator on institution letterhead. Orders will be billed at individual rate until proof of status is received. Foreign air speed delivery is included in all *Clinics* subscription prices. All prices are subject to change without notice. POSTMASTER: Send address changes to *Critical Care Clinics*, Elsevier Periodicals Customer Service, 11830 Westline Industrial Drive, St. Louis, MO 63146. **Customer Service: 1-800-654-2452 (US). From outside of the US, call 1-314-447-8871. Fax: 1-314-447-8029. E-mail: journalscustomerservice-usa@elsevier.com (for print support) or journalsonlinesupport-usa@elsevier.com (for online support).**

Reprints. For copies of 100 or more of articles in this publication, please contact the Commercial Reprints Department, Elsevier Inc., 360 Park Avenue South, New York, NY 10010-1710. Tel.: 212-633-3813; Fax: 212-462-1935; E-mail: reprints@elsevier.com.

Critical Care Clinics is also published in Spanish by Editorial Inter-Medica, Junin 917, 1er A, 1113, Buenos Aires, Argentina.

Critical Care Clinics is covered in *MEDLINE/PubMed (Index Medicus), EMBASE/Excerpta Medica, Current Concepts/Clinical Medicine, ISI/BIOMED, and Chemical Abstracts.*

Printed and bound by CPI Group (UK) Ltd, Croydon, CR0 4YY

Transferred to digital print 2012

Contributors

CONSULTING EDITOR

RICHARD W. CARLSON, MD, PhD
Chairman Emeritus, Director, Medical Intensive Care Unit, Department of Medicine, Maricopa Medical Center; Professor, University of Arizona College of Medicine; Professor, Department of Medicine, Mayo Graduate School of Medicine, Phoenix, Arizona

GUEST EDITOR

ROBERT C. HYZY, MD
Associate Professor, University of Michigan, Ann Arbor, Michigan

AUTHORS

NATHAN E. BRUMMEL, MD
Clinical Fellow, Division of Allergy, Pulmonary, and Critical Care Medicine, Department of Medicine; Department of Medicine, Center for Health Services Research, Vanderbilt University School of Medicine; Geriatric Research, Education and Clinical Center (GRECC) Service, Department of Veterans Affairs Medical Center, Tennessee Valley Healthcare System, Nashville, Tennessee

CAROL CHENOWETH, MD
Professor of Medicine and Hospital Epidemiologist, Division of Infectious Diseases, Departments of Internal Medicine and Infection Control and Epidemiology, University of Michigan Health System, Ann Arbor, Michigan

TIMOTHY D. GIRARD, MD, MSCI
Assistant Professor of Medicine, Division of Allergy, Pulmonary, and Critical Care Medicine, Department of Medicine; Department of Medicine, Center for Health Services Research, Vanderbilt University School of Medicine; Geriatric Research, Education and Clinical Center (GRECC) Service, Department of Veterans Affairs Medical Center, Tennessee Valley Healthcare System; Department of Medicine, Center for Quality of Aging, Vanderbilt University School of Medicine, Nashville, Tennessee

ROBERT C. HYZY, MD
Associate Professor, University of Michigan, Ann Arbor, Michigan

MARIN H. KOLLEF, MD
Professor of Medicine, Washington University School of Medicine, St. Louis, Missouri

JOHN P. KRESS, MD
Section of Pulmonary and Critical Care, Department of Medicine, University of Chicago, Chicago, Illinois

ANUPAM KUMAR, MD
Chief Medical Resident, Department of Medicine, Hartford Hospital, University of Connecticut Health Center, Farmington, Connecticut

MARK L. METERSKY, MD
Division of Pulmonary and Critical Care Medicine, University of Connecticut Health Center, Farmington, Connecticut

JAMES M. O'BRIEN JR, MD, MSc
Medical Director, Quality and Patient Safety, Riverside Methodist Hospital, Columbus, Ohio

PETER J. PRONOVOST, MS, PhD
Director, The Armstrong Institute for Patient Safety and Quality; Professor, The Department of Anesthesiology and Critical Care Medicine, Johns Hopkins University School of Medicine; The Department of Health Policy and Management, Johns Hopkins Bloomberg School of Public Health, Johns Hopkins University School of Nursing, Johns Hopkins Carey Business School, Baltimore, Maryland

ALAN D. RAVITZ, MS, PE
Program Manager–Biomedical Systems, The Johns Hopkins University Applied Physics Laboratory, Johns Hopkins University, Laurel, Maryland

MARK ROMIG, MD
Assistant Professor, The Department of Anesthesiology and Critical Care Medicine, Johns Hopkins University School of Medicine, Baltimore, Maryland

ROMMEL SAGANA, MD
Assistant Professor, University of Michigan, Ann Arbor, Michigan

SANJAY SAINT, MD, MPH
Director and VA/UM Patient Safety Enhancement Program Associate Chief of Medicine; Ann Arbor VA Medical Center George Dock Professor of Internal Medicine, University of Michigan Medical School, Ann Arbor, Michigan

ADAM SAPIRSTEIN, MD
The Armstrong Institute for Patient Safety and Quality; Associate Professor, The Department of Anesthesiology and Critical Care Medicine, Johns Hopkins University School of Medicine, Baltimore, Maryland

DAMON C. SCALES, MD, PhD
Interdepartmental Division of Critical Care, University of Toronto; Department of Critical Care Medicine, Sunnybrook Health Sciences Centre, Toronto, Ontario, Canada

ANDREW F. SHORR, MD, MPH
Associate Professor of Medicine, Georgetown University School of Medicine; Washington Hospital Center, Washington, DC

STEVEN P. TROPELLO, MD, MS
Senior Research Fellow, The Armstrong Institute for Patient Safety and Quality, Johns Hopkins University School of Medicine, Baltimore, Maryland

SAM R. WATSON, MSA, MA, CPPS
Executive Director, Michigan Health Association Keystone Centre, Lansing, Michigan

MARYA D. ZILBERBERG, MD, MPH
Adjunct Associate Professor, University of Massachusetts School of Public Health and Health Sciences, Amherst, Massachusetts; EviMed Research Group, LLC, Goshen, Massachusetts

Contents

Preface: Enhancing the Quality of Care in the Intensive Care Unit ix

Robert C. Hyzy

Achieving Zero Central Line–associated Bloodstream Infection Rates in Your Intensive Care Unit 1

Rommel Sagana and Robert C. Hyzy

Central line–associated bloodstream infection (CLABSI) is one of the most common health care–associated infections in the United States. The costs associated with CLABSIs include an estimated 28,000 deaths in the intensive care unit and up to $2.3 billion annually. Best practice guidelines, checklists, and establishing a culture of safety in hospitals are all initiatives designed to reduce the rate of CLABSI to zero.

Preventing *Clostridium Difficile* Infection in the Intensive Care Unit 11

Marya D. Zilberberg and Andrew F. Shorr

Clostridium difficile is a formidable problem in the twenty-first century. Because of injudicious use of antibiotics, the emergence of the hypervirulent epidemic strain of this organism has been difficult to contain. The NAP1/BI/027 strain causes more-severe disease than other widely prevalent strains and affects patients who were not traditionally thought to be at risk for *Clostridium difficile* infection. Critically ill patients remain at high risk for this pathogen, and preventive measures, such as meticulous contact precautions, hand hygiene, environmental disinfection, and, most importantly, antibiotic stewardship, are the cornerstones of mitigation in the intensive care unit.

Preventing Catheter-Associated Urinary Tract Infections in the Intensive Care Unit 19

Carol Chenoweth and Sanjay Saint

Urinary tract infection remains one of the most common healthcare-associated infections in the intensive care unit and predominantly occurs in patients with indwelling urinary catheters. Duration of catheterization is the most important risk factor for developing catheter-associated urinary tract infection (CAUTI). General strategies for preventing CAUTI include measures such as adherence to hand hygiene. Targeted strategies for preventing CAUTI include limiting the use and duration of urinary catheters, using aseptic technique for catheter insertion, and adhering to proper catheter care. Anti-infective catheters may be considered in some settings. Successful implementation of these measures has decreased urinary catheter use and CAUTI.

Ventilator-associated Complications, Including Infection-related Complications: The Way Forward 33

Marin H. Kollef

Acute respiratory failure represents the most common condition requiring admission to an adult intensive care unit. Ventilator-associated pneumonia

(VAP) has been used as a marker of quality for patients with respiratory failure. Hospital-based process-improvement initiatives to prevent VAP have been successfully used. The use of ventilator-associated complications (VACs) has been proposed as an objective marker to assess the quality of care for this patient population. The use of evidence-based bundles targeting the reduction of VACs, as well as the conduct of prospective studies showing that VACs are preventable complications, are reasonable first-steps in addressing this important clinical problem.

Preventing Delirium in the Intensive Care Unit 51

Nathan E. Brummel and Timothy D. Girard

Delirium in the intensive care unit (ICU) is exceedingly common, and risk factors for delirium among the critically ill are nearly ubiquitous. Addressing modifiable risk factors including sedation management, deliriogenic medications, immobility, and sleep disruption can help to prevent and reduce the duration of this deadly syndrome. The ABCDE approach to critical care is a bundled approach that clinicians can implement for many patients treated in their ICUs to prevent the adverse outcomes associated with delirium and critical illness.

Sedation and Mobility: Changing the Paradigm 67

John P. Kress

A large fraction of intensive care unit (ICU) patients with respiratory failure who survive their critical illness leave the hospital with substantial neuromuscular weakness. In light of this reality, a shift in the approach to critical care management has begun. This viewpoint has broadened the perspective of ICU care providers beyond the narrow goal of leaving the ICU alive to a broader notion focused on minimizing the complications that accompany the inherent noxious nature of ICU care. Mobilization of mechanically ventilated patients is feasible, safe, and carries the potential for tremendous benefit for our patients.

Improving Intensive Care Unit Quality Using Collaborative Networks 77

Sam R. Watson and Damon C. Scales

Collaborative networks of intensive care units can help promote a quality-improvement agenda across an entire system or region. Proposed advantages include targeting a greater number of patients, sharing of resources, and common measurement systems for audit and feedback or benchmarking. This review focuses on elements that are essential for the success and sustainability of these collaborative networks, using as examples networks in Michigan and Ontario. More research is needed to understand the mechanisms through which collaborative networks lead to improved care delivery and to demonstrate their cost-effectiveness in comparison with other approaches to system-level quality improvement.

Does Value-Based Purchasing Enhance Quality of Care and Patient Outcomes in the ICU? 91

James M. O'Brien Jr, Anupam Kumar, and Mark L. Metersky

As health care expenditures increase, payers, including the Centers for Medicare and Medicaid Services, are moving away from reimbursement based on types and volume of services to an emphasis on quality of provided care, an approach called value-based purchasing (VBP). Because it is tied to reimbursement, VBP creates economic motivation to measure and improve care. VBP is proceeding without high-level evidence supporting its effectiveness in improving health care quality. Rising health care costs, however, make VBP an attractive approach for curtailing costs and emphasizing improved quality, and VBP is likely to become a more prevalent mechanism of reimbursement for providers and facilities.

Enhancing the Quality of Care in the Intensive Care Unit: A Systems Engineering Approach **113**

Steven P. Tropello, Alan D. Ravitz, Mark Romig, Peter J. Pronovost, and Adam Sapirstein

This article presents an overview of systems engineering and describes common core principles found in systems engineering methodologies. The Patient Care Program Acute Care Initiative collaboration between the Armstrong Institute of the Johns Hopkins School of Medicine and the Gordon and Betty Moore Foundation, which will use systems engineering to reduce patient harm in the intensive care unit, is introduced. Specific examples of applying a systems engineering approach to the Patient Care Program Acute Care Initiative are presented.

Index **125**

Enhancing the Quality of Care in the ICU

CRITICAL CARE CLINICS

FORTHCOMING ISSUES

April 2013
Pediatric Critical Care
Margaret Parker, MD, *Guest Editor*

July 2013
Life-Threatening Infections: Part 1
Anand Kumar, MD, *Guest Editor*

October 2013
Life-Threatening Infections: Part 2
Anand Kumar, MD, *Guest Editor*

RECENT ISSUES

October 2012
Toxicology
James A. Kruse, MD, *Guest Editor*

July 2012
Nonmalignant Hematology
Robert I. Parker, MD, *Guest Editor*

April 2012
Cardiopulmonary Resuscitation
Wanchun Tang, MD, Master CCM, FAHA, *Guest Editor*

Preface

Enhancing the Quality of Care in the Intensive Care Unit

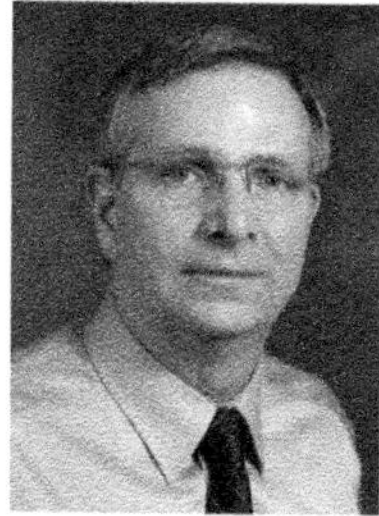

Robert C. Hyzy, MD
Guest Editor

At some point everyone working in the area of quality improvement in medicine cites "To Err is Human" as the seminal moment when the medical field decided to focus its attention on decreasing medical errors and enhancing the quality of care delivered. Yet, medicine faces unique challenges which are unlike those of other "industries" whose efforts in the area of error reduction and quality improvement antedated those of medicine. The Six Sigma airline industry analogy, while worthy, is insufficient in that it fails to recognize the critical element of practice culture in determining outcomes. Put more simply, it is not a just about the checklist. As Heraclitus said, "no man steps in the same river twice." However, this should never serve to rationalize poor practice culture, frequently justified as "my patients are different." No successful study in the intensive care unit (ICU) can improve the quality of care delivered to patients without some ability to regulate interpersonal interactions. Subsequently, the ability to translate these behavioral changes to the bedside as a part of routine care on a daily basis becomes the real challenge, be it compliance with lung protective ventilation, sedation holidays, discontinuing central lines or urinary catheters, and so on. The success of the Michigan Keystone ICU collaborative is owed to the many nursing and physician leaders who served to champion the behavioral changes required to change the process of care in their ICUs. Change is not only possible, it is sustainable. Medicine has progressed to a different epoch of care from when the Institute of Medicine published "To Err is Human." ICU quality has moved forward, sometimes fitfully (tight glycemic control), at other times forcefully (early mobility), but forward nevertheless. When asked by the editors of *Critical Care Clinics* if I would be willing to edit an edition on improving the quality of care in the ICU, I greedily accepted. It has been a privilege to interact and become friends with many of the most outstanding investigators working in the ICU to move our practice forward. I was honored they accepted my invitation to

Crit Care Clin 29 (2013) ix–x
http://dx.doi.org/10.1016/j.ccc.2012.11.001
criticalcare.theclinics.com

make a contribution. I believe this collection offers the reader a thorough and concise primer on where we are in ICU quality improvement and where we are headed.

Robert C. Hyzy, MD
University of Michigan
3916 Taubman Center
Ann Arbor, MI 48109, USA

E-mail address:
rhyzy@umich.edu

Achieving Zero Central Line–associated Bloodstream Infection Rates in Your Intensive Care Unit

Rommel Sagana, MD, Robert C. Hyzy, MD*

KEYWORDS

• CLABSI • HAI • BSI • VAP

KEY POINTS

- Central line–associated bloodstream infection (CLABSI) is one of the most common health care–associated infections in the United States.
- The costs associated with CLABSIs include an estimated 28,000 deaths in the intensive care unit and up to $2.3 billion annually.
- Best practice guidelines, checklists, and establishing a culture of safety in hospitals are all initiatives designed to reduce the rate of CLABSI to zero.

Health care–associated infections (HAIs) are among the most common adverse events that occur during hospital admissions. Bloodstream infections (BSIs) are an important cause of morbidity and mortality with an estimated 250,000 cases occurring each year in the United States.[1] Most of these infections are primarily associated with intravascular catheters.[2] Primary BSIs from the use of intravenous catheters comprise most of the nosocomial BSIs reported to the National Nosocomial Infection Surveillance (NNIS) system of the Centers for Disease Control and Prevention (CDC).[3]

A prospective analysis from the Surveillance and Control of Pathogens of Epidemiologic Importance (SCOPE) database reported the incidence of nosocomial BSI to be 60 cases per 10,000 hospital admissions. Intravascular devices were the most common predisposing factor. A central venous catheter was in place in 72% of cases.[4] Central line–associated BSIs (CLABSIs), occur up to 80,000 times per year, resulting in 28,000 deaths among patients in intensive care units (ICUs). The average cost of care for a patient with this type of infection is approximately $45,000, therefore the annual cost could be as high as $2.3 billion annually.[5]

Although quality control interventions in many areas of ICU care have been studied, the idea of integrating quality indicators with groups of interventions known as bundles has been validated in the ICU most successfully with CLABSI: in the Michigan Health

University of Michigan, 3916 Taubman Center, Ann Arbor, MI 48109, USA
* Corresponding author.
E-mail address: rhyzy@umich.edu

Crit Care Clin 29 (2013) 1–9
http://dx.doi.org/10.1016/j.ccc.2012.10.003 criticalcare.theclinics.com
0749-0704/13/$ – see front matter

and Hospitals Keystone ICU project, Pronovost and colleagues[6] showed that simple and inexpensive interventions, grouped now famously as a checklist, could reduce the rate of a nosocomial infection to a median rate of zero across a state. The study intervention recommended 5 evidence-based procedures recommended by the CDC that were identified as having the greatest effect on the rate of catheter-related BSIs and the lowest barriers to implementation.[7] The recommended procedures were hand washing, using full-barrier precautions during the insertion of central venous catheters, cleaning the skin with chlorhexidine, avoiding the femoral site if possible, and removing unnecessary catheters.

To implement these strategies, clinicians were first educated about practices to control infection and harm resulting from catheter-related BSIs. Central line carts with necessary supplies were created. A checklist was used to ensure adherence to infection-control practices. Providers were stopped (in nonemergency situations) if these practices were not being followed. The removal of catheters was discussed at daily rounds and teams received feedback regarding the numbers and rates of catheter-related BSI at monthly and quarterly meetings, respectively. The study coordinators made sure chlorhexidine was stocked in the participating hospitals before initiation of the study.

One-hundred and three out of 108 participating Michigan ICUs reported data. The median rate of catheter-related BSI per 1000 catheter days decreased from 2.7 infections at baseline to 0 at 3 months after implementation of the study intervention ($P \leq .002$). The mean rate per 1000 catheter days decreased from 7.7 at baseline to 1.4 at 16 to 18 months of follow-up ($P \leq .002$). There was a significant decrease in infection rates from baseline, with incidence-rate ratios continuously decreasing from 0.62 (95% confidence interval [CI], 0.47–0.81) at 0 to 3 months after implementation of the intervention to 0.34 (95% CI, 0.23–0.50) at 16 to 18 months.[6]

Since that landmark study, there have been additional efforts to clarify guidelines that provide comprehensive recommendations for detecting and preventing HAIs. In 2008, the Society for Healthcare Epidemiology of America/Infectious Diseases Society of America published guidelines containing strategies to detect and prevent CLABSI. Recommendations for implementing prevention and monitoring CLABSI infection rates were given along with the criteria for grading the strength of the recommendation using Grades of Recommendation, Assessment, Development and Evaluation (GRADE) criteria and quality of evidence presented (**Table 1**).[8]

Basic practices for prevention and monitoring of CLABSI were recommended for all acute care hospitals. Specific recommendations before insertion of the catheter are shown in **Box 1**.

Further recommendations that are applicable after insertion of the catheter are shown in **Box 2**.

The practice of using bundles or checklists has become widely implemented. In addition to treatment of sepsis and prevention of CLABSI, the reduction of ventilator-associated pneumonia (VAP) in the ICU involves another order set that has been bundled. For example, again in Michigan, Berenholtz and colleagues[9] implemented a multifaceted intervention to improve compliance with 5 evidence-based recommendations for mechanically ventilated patients and to prevent VAP. Compared with baseline, VAP rates decreased during all observation periods, with incidence-rate ratios of 0.51 (95% CI, 0.41–0.64) at 16 to 18 months after implementation and 0.29 (95% CI, 0.24–0.34) at 28 to 30 months after implementation. An important observation noted in this study and in other studies involving bundles is that, although the individual recommendations may not be strong in producing the desired outcome, taken as a whole, the bundle achieves significant and sustained results.

Table 1
Strength of recommendation and quality of evidence

Category/Grade	Definition
Strength of Recommendation	
A	Good evidence to support a recommendation for use
B	Moderate evidence to support a recommendation for use
C	Poor evidence to support a recommendation
Quality of Evidence	
I	Evidence from ≥1 properly randomized, controlled trial
II	Evidence from ≥1 well-designed clinical trial, without randomization; from cohort or case control analytical studies (preferably from >1 center); from multiple time series; or from dramatic results of uncontrolled experiments
III	Evidence from opinions of respected authorities, based on clinical experience, descriptive studies, or reports from expert committees

Data from the Canadian Task Force on the Periodic Health; and *From* Brown J, Doloresco F III, Mylotte JM. Never events: not every hospital-acquired infection is preventable. Clin Infect Dis 2009;49:743–6.

Closer evaluation of these improvements also reveals a consistent trend in the rate of quality improvement. These trends develop over several years. Our own institution's experience with CLABSI bundles shows a significant reduction of CLABSI rates over a period of 3 years.[10] A possible explanation for this phenomenon involves not only evaluating the results of the implemented bundles but also the effect of those changes on the safety culture on the participating institutions.

Culture of safety was placed on the health care research agenda by the Institute of Medicine in the 1999 report, "To Err is Human."[11] From an anthropologic perspective, assessing culture involves careful and time-consuming observation of norms, beliefs, values, and rituals. Social scientists often forego the deeper cultural assessment and opt for the more efficient technique of climate assessment. Climate assessment involves administering questionnaires to obtain a surface reading of the norms and behaviors of a given group. Safety climate has been widely researched in other industries[12,13] in which it predicts unsafe[14] and safety-specific behaviors,[15] injury rates,[16] and accidents.[17]

Box 1
Prior insertion: basic practices for prevention and monitoring of CLABSI; recommended for all acute care hospitals

1. Educate health care personnel involved in the insertion, care, and maintenance of central venous catheters (CVCs) about CLABSI prevention (A-II).
2. Use a catheter checklist to ensure adherence to infection prevention practices at the time of CVC insertion (B-II).
3. Perform hand hygiene before catheter insertion or manipulation (B-II).
4. Avoid using the femoral vein for central venous access in adult patients (A-I).
5. Use an all-inclusive catheter cart or kit (B-II).
6. Use maximal sterile barrier precautions during CVC insertion (A-I).
7. Use a chlorhexidine-based antiseptic for skin preparations in patients more than 2 months old (A-I).

Box 2
After insertion: basic practices for prevention and monitoring of CLABSI; recommended for all acute care hospitals

1. Disinfect catheter hubs, needleless connectors, and injection ports before accessing the catheter (B-II).
2. Remove nonessential catheters (A-II).
3. Specific care for nontunneled CVCs.
4. Replace administration sets not used for blood, blood products, or lipids at intervals no longer than 96 hours (A-II).
5. Perform surveillance for CLABSI (B-II).
6. Use antimicrobial ointments for hemodialysis catheter insertion sites (A-I).

The terms culture and climate are used interchangeably; however, in health care, safety climate is better defined as the consensus of shared perceptions regarding patient safety norms and behaviors by frontline workers in a given clinical area. Studies have linked safety climate to clinical and operational outcomes in addition to showing that safety climate is responsive to interventions.[18,19] In 2011, a large-scale study evaluated the impact of a comprehensive unit-based safety program (CUSP) on safety climate in the statewide Michigan Keystone ICU Project.[20] The study was a prospective cohort designed to improve quality of care and safety culture by implementing and evaluating patient safety interventions in participating ICUs. A validated safety attitudes questionnaire (SAQ)[21] was given in 2004 and again in 2006 to assess improvement. The SAQ addressed perceptions of management, teamwork climate, job satisfaction, stress recognition, and working conditions. The safety climate scale is calculated using 7 items and a 5-point Likert scale, from disagree strongly to agree strongly. A score of less than 60% was in the needs-improvement zone and a discrepancy greater than or equal to 10 points in pre-post scores was needed to describe a difference.

Before administering the SAQ, 5 sequential steps were implemented over several months. In step 1, teams were educated on the science of safety and were given tools to educate their staff. Step 2 involved having teams identify, prioritize, and eliminate patient safety hazards in their ICU. In step 3, teams were instructed to partner with a senior leader within their organization. The senior leader's role was to round monthly with the staff, review safety hazards, ensure the team had resources and political support to implement interventions that reduced safety risks, and hold the team accountable for mitigating hazards. In step 4, teams were encouraged to learn from 1 defect per month using a structured form[22] that asked what happened, why it happened, what was done to reduce risk, and how it was confirmed that risk was reduced. Step 5 implemented tools to improve communication among caregivers in the ICU.

The study also introduced a multifaceted intervention of evidence-based prevention practices to reduce catheter-related BSIs,[13] a daily-goals checklist to improve communication among clinicians in the ICU,[23] and a multifaceted intervention of evidence-based practices to reduce VAP.[24]

Seventy-one ICUs completed the study. Overall mean safety climate scores significantly improved from 42.5% (2004) to 52.2% (2006) (*P*<.001). In 2004, 87% of participating ICUs were in the need-improvement zone, whereas in 2006 only 47% were in this range. This study was the first to show large-scale improvements in safety climate among diverse organizations. The next phase of the study involves linking improved climate scores with clinical and operational outcomes in the ICU. It can be inferred that, although outcomes are important, organization of care leads to better care outcomes both directly and indirectly as the overall safety climate of an institution improves.

CLABSIs, along with surgical site infections (SSIs), catheter-associated urinary tract infections (CAUTIs), and VAP, account for 75% of all HAIs.[25] HAIs are one of the most common complications involving hospital care and are a leading cause of death in the United States.[26] HAIs affected an estimated 5% of hospitalized patients in the United States in 2002.[25] In 2002, HAIs accounted for 1.7 million infections and an estimated 99,000 deaths, most of which resulted from CLABSIs and VAP.[27]

The health and economic impacts of HAIs are extensive.[28] The impact of CLABSI in particular includes an 18% increase in the probability of mortality and a 13-day increase in ICU length of stay (LOS).[28,29] There is a wide range of estimates regarding the costs related to CLABSI. A 2007 review of the literature identified costs per CLABSI to range from $2820 to $13,000, with a mean of $10,531 in 2005 dollars. This cost is equivalent to $12,208 in 2010 US dollars.[30] A study of the additional marginal cost associated with these infections in Calgary, Canada, found even higher costs. ICU-acquired BSIs cost an additional $25,155 Canadian dollars per case, which is equal to $19,199 in 2010 US dollars.[31] Estimates that include the extra LOS in a hospital resulting from CLABSI was approximately $22,939 in 2003 US dollars.[32] Earlier studies estimated that total hospital costs were as high as $56,167 after adjusting for demographics and severity of disease.[33]

Certain HAIs are preventable but, as prevention efforts become more defined, there remains a lack of evidence of a strong return of investment for hospitals and health care payers in preventing these infections. This lack of evidence presents a potential obstacle in advancing efforts to prevent infections.[34] Current reimbursement structures in the US health care system do not provide incentives to reduce HAIs.[35] Payment incentives for hospitals, on either a per-case or a fee-for-service basis, typically encourage volume rather than outcomes. This system is changing with a movement toward quality-based purchasing.

The term business case in health care is used to describe a situation in which the organization investing in an intervention gains a positive return on an investment within a defined period of time and using an accepted discount rate.[36] A business case in health care may be based on improvements in organizational function and sustainability that have long-term benefits.[37]

A recent study by Waters and colleagues[36] calculated the results of a patient safety intervention in the form of cost-effectiveness analysis presented as the cost per infection averted. It also conducted an economic cost-benefit analysis from the hospital perspective for the implementation of a patient safety initiative. The study was part of the Michigan Keystone ICU Patient Safety Program. A key component of the program included a CUSP that had interventions to improve safety culture, teamwork, and communication, a daily goals sheet, and other communication tools. The study also included specific interventions to improve compliance with evidence-based care to reduce CLABSIs and VAP that were derived using the Johns Hopkins Quality and Safety Research Group (QSRG) method for translating evidence into practice.

A total of 108 ICUs in the state participated, with 103 ICUs reporting data. The mean rate of incidence of CLABI decreased from 7.7 per 1000 catheter days at baseline to 1.3 at 16 to 18 months' follow-up. The rate decreased to 1.1 per 1000 catheter days at 34 to 36 months' follow-up. The median rates for CLABSI decreased from 2.7 at baseline to 0 at 16 to 18 months and beyond.[6,38]

For the economic analysis, a subsample of 6 hospitals that participated in the main Keystone ICU project was selected. Incremental operational costs of the Keystone ICU project, which include salary of hospital staff, costs of equipment, supplies, laboratory, and drugs, were calculated using activity-based costing techniques.[39,40] These techniques use interviews to determine the distribution of individuals' time among the program's principal activities and assigns costs through these activities. These interviews included the following staff categories: ICU director, intensivists, other physicians, ICU nurses, Keystone ICU team leaders, senior hospital administrators, infection prevention staff, and pharmacists. The principal method for enhanced accuracy using this method is that indirect costs are allocated in proportion to personnel time, which more closely mirrors the consumption of resources than does allocation based on volume.[41]

To calculate the number of CLABSI cases averted by the intervention in each hospital, the median and mean CLABSI rates expressed as the number of cases per 1000 days of exposure on the catheter per 3-month interval were extracted from the published articles describing the Keystone ICU Patient Safety Program.[6,38] Applying the mean rate of decline in number of CLABSIs, on average, 29.9 CLABSIs were averted annually at each of the 6 hospitals by fiscal year 2008. VAP rates also decreased from a mean rate of 6.9 per 1000 ventilator days at baseline to 2.4 at 30 months after implementation. Again, applying the mean rate to decline to the number of ventilator days in each ICU showed that the interventions averted 18 cases of VAP at each hospital on an annual basis. Summing the CLABSI and VAP rates, the interventions averted 47.9 infections per hospital per year. The cost of the interventions was $3375 per infection averted, measured in 2007 dollars.

The cost of the intervention is modest compared with the cost associated with infection. In the United States, the extra hospital costs associated with each episode of CLABSI range from $12,208 to $56,167.[30,33] Estimates of the total financial burden attributable to HAIs range from $4.5 billion to $45 billion annually.[25,32] The findings from the Waters and colleagues[36] study likely underestimate the overall savings associated with preventing HAIs. People who develop complications that require an extended stay in an ICU generally have longer stays in a rehabilitation facility, have a greater use of home health services, and have longer absences from work.

In addition to the financial incentives of preventing CLABSI infections, there is also the mortality benefit associated with decreasing infection rates. The CDC estimates that there are 250,000 cases of CLABSI in US hospitals, with an attributable mortality of 12% to 25%.[5,31,42] Applying this rate to the interventions in Michigan suggests that between 3.4 and 7.2 deaths from CLABSI per hospital have been prevented annually by the Keystone ICU project.

As part of a national effort to reduce HAIs, the Department of Health and Human Services (HHS) launched the HHS Action Plan to reduce Prevent Healthcare-Associated Infections in 2009. As part of this action plan, the Agency for Healthcare Research and Quality (AHRQ) increased the support and scope of a project funded in 2008 designed to reduce CLABSIs. This project was titled On the Cusp: Stop BSI.[43] This project was designed to apply the CUSP to improve the culture of patient safety and implement evidence-based best practices to reduce the risk of infection.[43] Final data from this project are pending but the initial results are reported to be encouraging.

Health care institutions have entered a pay-for-performance era, with emphasis on the prevention of hospital-acquired infections. In 2008, the Centers for Medicare and Medicaid Services (CMS) stopped paying hospitals for cases involving so-called never events,[44] which are cases involving potentially preventable adverse events including

CAUTIs, SSI, and CLABSIs. Organizational bundles are the current tools designed to prevent infection from catheter insertion to removal. However, as shown in Keystone ICU safety culture animates checklists. Without creating a culture of safety, checklists and bundles, no matter how well intentioned or evidenced based, are destined to fail.

REFERENCES

1. Pittet D, Li N, Woolson RF, et al. Microbiological factors influencing the outcome of nosocomial blood stream infections: a 6-year validated, population-based model. Clin Infect Dis 1997;24:1068.
2. Wisplinghoff H, Bischoff T, Tallent SM, et al. Nosocomial bloodstream infections in US hospitals: analysis of 24,179 cases from a prospective nationwide surveillance study. Clin Infect Dis 2004;39:309.
3. Martone WJ, Gaynes RP, Horac TC, et al. National Nosocomial Infections Surveillance (NNIS) semiannual report, May 1995. A report from the National Nosocomial Infections Surveillance (NNIS) System. Am J Infect Control 1995;23:377.
4. Centers for Disease Control and Prevention (CDC). Vital signs: central line-associated blood stream infections—United States, 2001, 2008, and 2009. MMWR Morb Mortal Wkly Rep 2011;60:243.
5. O'Grady NP, Alexander M, Dellinger EP, et al. Guidelines for the prevention of intravascular catheter-related infections. MMWR Recomm Rep 2002;51(RR–10): 1–29.
6. Pronovost P, Needham D, Berenholtz S, et al. An intervention to decrease catheter-related bloodstream infections in the ICU. N Engl J Med 2006;355(26): 2725–32.
7. Mermel LA. Prevention of intravascular catheter-related infections. Ann Intern Med 2000;132:391–402.
8. Supplemental article: SHEA/IDSA Practice Recommendation. Marschall J, Mermel LA, Classen D, et al. Strategies to prevent central line-associated bloodstream infections in acute care hospitals. Infect Control Hosp Epidemiol 2008;29: S22–30.
9. Berenholtz SM, Pham JC, Thompson DA, et al. Collaborative cohort study of an intervention to reduce ventilator-associated pneumonia in the intensive care unit. Infect Control Hosp Epidemiol 2011;32(4):305–14.
10. Shuman EK, Washer LL, Arndt JL, et al. Analysis of central line-associated bloodstream infections in the intensive care unit after implementation of central line bundles. Infect Control Hosp Epidemiol 2010;31(5):551–3.
11. Kohn L, Corrigan J, Donaldson M (Eds): Creating safety systems in health care organizations. In: To Err is Human: Building a Safer Health System. Washington, DC: National Academy Press; 1999. p. 155–202.
12. Zohar D. A group-level model of safety climate: testing the effect of group climate microaccidents in manufacturing jobs. J Appl Psychol 2000;85:587–96.
13. Cheyne A, Cox S, Oliver A, et al. Modeling safety climate in the prediction of levels of safety activity. Work Stress 1998;12:255–71.
14. Cooper MD, Phillips RA. Exploratory analysis of the safety climate and safety behavior relationship. J Safety Res 2004;35:497–512.
15. Zohar D, Livne Y, Tenne-Gazit O, et al. Healthcare climate: a framework for measuring and improving patient safety. Crit Care Med 2007;35:1312–7.
16. Barling J, Loughlin C, Kelloway EK. Developing and test of a model linking safety-specific transformational leadership and occupational safety. J Appl Psychol 2002;87:488–96.

17. Hoffman DA, Stetzer A. A cross-level investigation of factors influencing unsafe behavior and accidents. Person Psychol 1996;49:307–39.
18. Pronovost P, Weast B, Rosenstein B, et al. Implementing and validating a comprehensive unit-based safety program. J Patient Saf 2005;1:33–40.
19. Defontes J, Surbida S. Preoperative safety briefing project. Perm J 2004;8:21–7.
20. Sexton JB, Berenholtz SM, Goeschel CA, et al. Assessing and improving safety climate in a large cohort on intensive care units. Crit Care Med 2011;39: 934–9.
21. Sexton JB, Helmreich RL, Neilands TB, et al. The Safety Attitudes Questionnaire: psychometric properties benchmarking data, and emerging research. BMC Health Serv Res 2006;6:44.
22. Pronovost PJ, Holzmueller CG, Martinez E, et al. A practical tool to learn from defects in patient care. Jt Comm J Qual Patient Saf 2006;32:102–8.
23. Pronovost P, Berenholtz S, Dorman T, et al. Improving communication in the ICU using daily goals. J Crit Care 2003;18:71–5.
24. Berenholtz SM, Milanovich S, Faircloth A, et al. Improving care for the ventilated patient. Jt Comm J Qual Saf 2004;30:195–204.
25. Department of Health and Human Services. HHS action plan to prevent healthcare-associated infections. Washington, DC: US Department of Health and Human Services; 2009. Available at: http://hhs.gov/ash/initiatives/hai. Accessed June 1, 2009.
26. Klevens RM, Edwards JR, Richards CL Jr, et al. Estimating health care-associated infections and deaths in U.S. hospitals, 2002. Public Health Rep 2007;122:160–6.
27. Hidron AI, Edwards JR, Patel J, et al. NHSN annual update: antimicrobial-resistant pathogens associated with healthcare-associated infections: annual summary of data reported to the National Healthcare Safety Network at the Centers for Disease Control and Prevention, 2006-2007. Infect Control Hosp Epidemiol 2008;29:996–1011.
28. Pittet D, Tarara D, Wenzel RP. Nosocomial bloodstream infections in critically ill patients. Excess length of stay, extra costs, and attributable mortality. JAMA 1994;271:1598–601.
29. Heiselman D. Nosocomial bloodstream infections in the critically ill. Ann Intern Med 1994;272:1819–20.
30. Halton K, Graves N. Economic evaluation and catheter-related bloodstream infections. Emerg Infect Dis 2007;13:815–23.
31. Laupland KB, Lee H, Gregson DB, et al. Cost of intensive care unit-acquired bloodstream infections. J Hosp Infect 2006;63:124–32.
32. Scott RD. The direct medical costs of healthcare-associated infections in U.S. hospitals and the benefit of prevention. Available at: http://www.cdc.gov/ncidod/dhqp/pdf/Scott_CostPaper.pdf. Accessed March 1, 2009.
33. Dimick JB, Pronovost PJ, Heitmiller RF, et al. Intensive care unit physician staffing is associated with decreased length of stay, hospital cost, and complications after esophageal resections. Crit Care Med 2001;29:753–8.
34. Galvin RS, Delbanco S, Milstein A, et al. Has the Leapfrog Group had an impact on the health care market? Health Aff (Millwood) 2005;24:228–33.
35. Coye MJ. No Toyotas in health care: why medical care has not evolved to meet patients' needs. Health Aff (Millwood) 2001;20:44–56.
36. Waters HR, Korn RK Jr, Colantuoni E, et al. The business case for quality: economic analysis of the Michigan Keystone Patient Safety Program in ICUs. Am J Med Qual 2011;26(5):333–9.

37. Leatherman S, Berwick D, Iles D, et al. The business case for quality: case studies and an analysis. Health Aff (Millwood) 2003;22:17–30.
38. Pronovost P, Goeschel CA, Colantuoni, et al. Sustaining reductions in catheter related blood stream infections in Michigan intensive care units: observational study. BMJ 2010;340:c309.
39. Canby J. Applying activity-based costing to healthcare settings. Healthc Financ Manage 1995;49:50–2, 54–6.
40. Waters HR, Abdallah H, Santillan D. Application of activity-based costing (ABC) for a Peruvian NGO healthcare provider. Int J Health Plann Manage 2001;16: 3–18.
41. Baker JJ. How activity-based costing works in health care. In: Activity-based costing and activity-based management for health care. (B. Macdonald, Ed.) Gaithersburg (MD): Jones & Bartlett Learning; 1998. p. 15–28.
42. Centers for Disease Control and Prevention. Reduction in central line-associated bloodstream infections among patients in intensive care units—Pennsylvania, April 2001-March 2005. MMWR Morb Mortal Wkly Rep 2005;54:1013–6.
43. Available at: http://www.onthecuspstophai.org/on-the-cuspstop-bsi/. Accessed September 30, 2008.
44. Brown J, Doloresco F III, Mylotte JM. Never events: not every hospital-acquired infection is preventable. Clin Infect Dis 2009;49:743–6.

Preventing *Clostridium Difficile* Infection in the Intensive Care Unit

Marya D. Zilberberg, MD, MPH[a,b,*], Andrew F. Shorr, MD, MPH[c,d]

KEYWORDS

• *Clostridium difficile* • Infectious diarrhea • ICU • Antibiotic stewardship

KEY POINTS

- *Clostridium difficile* is a formidable problem in the twenty-first century.
- Because of injudicious use of antibiotics, the emergence of the hypervirulent epidemic strain of this organism has been difficult to contain.
- The NAP1/BI/027 strain causes more severe disease than other widely prevalent strains and affects patients who had not been traditionally thought to be at risk for *C difficile* infection.
- Critically ill patients remain at high risk for this pathogen, and preventive measures, such as meticulous contact precautions, hand hygiene, environmental disinfection, and, most importantly, antibiotic stewardship, are the cornerstones of mitigation.
- The positive preliminary data for the role of probiotics in the intensive care unit population are intriguing, although their risk/benefit ratio requires further confirmation.

Identified as a pathogen in antibiotic-associated diarrhea in 1978, *Clostridium difficile* is a gram-positive spore-forming anaerobe. It is the leading cause of antibiotic-associated diarrhea, responsible for most health care–associated diarrheal illnesses. The severity of disease caused by *C difficile* may span the gamut from nuisance and mild abdominal discomfort to severe colitis, toxic megacolon, and death.

Over the past decade, *C difficile* has gained importance as a deadly pathogen. Beginning in the late 1990s, multiple groups noted that the epidemiology and outcomes of *C difficile* infection (CDI) in hospitals were evolving. A report from Pepin in 2004 documented a shocking 5-fold increase in the incidence of CDI in Quebec,

---

Disclosure: Dr Zilberberg has received consulting fees and research funding from ViroPharma, manufacturer of Vancocin; and Optimer, manufacturer of fidoxamicin. The content of this manuscript was presented in part at the Society of Critical Care Medicine 2012 annual meeting.
[a] Evi*Med* Research Group, LLC, PO Box 303, Goshen, MA 01032, USA; [b] University of Massachusetts School of Public Health and Health Sciences, Amherst, MA 01003, USA; [c] Washington Hospital Center, Washington, DC 20010, USA; [d] Georgetown University School of Medicine, Washington, DC, USA

* Corresponding author. Evi*Med* Research Group, LLC, PO Box 303, Goshen, MA 01032.
E-mail address: evimedgroup@gmail.com

Crit Care Clin 29 (2013) 11–18
http://dx.doi.org/10.1016/j.ccc.2012.10.006 criticalcare.theclinics.com
0749-0704/13/$ – see front matter

Canada, increasing from 36 to 156 cases per 100,000 population between 1992 and 2003.[1] This increase was accompanied by roughly a doubling of the proportion that exhibited severe and complicated disease. In the United States, similar developments were noted first in Pittsburgh, Pennsylvania, and then across the United States.[2] Sobering reports on the nationwide trends in CDI hospitalizations signaled a rapid doubling of CDI cases in U.S. hospitals between the mid 1990s and mid-2000s, with a similar 2-fold rise in case fatality.[3,4]

An investigation by the Centers for Disease Control and Prevention identified a new strain of *C difficile* named *NAP1/BI/027* (toxinotype III, North American pulsed-field gel electrophoresis type 1, polymerase chain reaction–ribotype 027 [NAP1/027]).[5] This strain, responsible for a substantial proportion of the new epidemic cases, has several features that explain its hypervirulent character: it is capable of producing approximately 20 times the amount of the toxins A and B than other clinically relevant strains, and its plentiful spores are more adherent and, therefore, more likely to linger in the gut, and are more suited to being transmitted through fomites.[6] Genetically, a deletion in the regulatory portion of the toxin-producing allele is present in the new strain, prompting exuberant and unchecked toxin overproduction. A binary toxin gene has also been identified, although its role remains a mystery. An important clinical feature of NAP1/BI/027 is its high level of fluoroquinolone resistance in vitro. Since the strain became evident in the early 2000s, it has been reported in most of the states in the United States, and in many locations abroad.

Several epidemiologic features of CDI now directly reflect this increased virulence. Namely, the disease it causes is more severe, exhibiting greater morbidity and mortality and resulting in a higher likelihood of the need for intensive care unit (ICU) care.[1,2,4,7–9] In addition, CDI now can afflict what were previously considered low-risk populations: the young, those without comorbidities, and persons without a history of exposure to antibiotics.[10]

The economic burden of CDI is not trivial, particularly among those who require hospitalization. Four studies examined the costs attributable to a CDI admission, and these estimates range from approximately $3000 to more than $15,000 per case in 2008.[11] This broad range of values is because of different methodologies used and research questions asked. Nonetheless, extrapolating these costs to the full complement of 2008 CDI hospitalizations hints at the staggering price tag that this infection carries. Namely, the range of total CDI acute hospitalization costs is between $1 and $4.8 billion.[11]

Although no study has specifically focused on CDI costs in the ICU, these critically ill patients are likely to incur an even higher cost from this complication. In a study of patients receiving 96 or more hours of mechanical ventilation or prolonged acute mechanical ventilation (PAMV), the authors noted an additional 6.1-day hospital length of stay and $10,355 in hospital costs among PAMV discharges with CDI.[12] The design, however, did not allow for the calculation of the attributable economic burden.

CDI EPIDEMIOLOGY IN THE ICU

The prevalence of CDI among the general hospitalized population is reported to be much less than 2%. McDonald and colleagues[3] reported that nationally in the United States, the annual volume of hospitalizations with CDI increased from 82,000 to 178,000 between 1996 and 2003. Similar reports based on the Nationwide Inpatient Sample documented a prevalence of CDI between 7 and 10 cases per 1000 hospitalizations in 2006, depending on the geographic region, or less than 1% of all adult acute hospitalizations.[4]

In the ICU, however, the proportion of patients with CDI is far higher, approaching 5% in some populations. Thus, in a single-center retrospective cohort enrolled before year 2000, Lawrence and colleagues[13] noted that 76 of 1872 critically ill patients had evidence of CDI, with roughly one-half developing it while in the ICU. The authors' group has examined the epidemiology and outcomes of CDI among patients on PAMV in the Nationwide Inpatient Sample, a database that is a 20% representative sample of all acute hospital discharges in the United States.[12] They found that in 2005, among the 64,910 PAMV discharges, 3468 (5.3%) had a concomitant International Classification of Disease, 9th Edition, Clinical Modification (ICD-9-CM) diagnosis of CDI, and its prevalence increased with age.

Risk factors for CDI in the ICU are largely similar to those found on a general ward. Bobo and colleagues,[14] in their timely review of CDI in the ICU, divided these risks into 3 categories: (1) perturbation of the intestinal flora/mucosa or immune system (eg, from exposures to antibiotics, proton pump inhibitors, chemotherapy), (2) environmental contamination, and (3) host factors. Although most of these factors are well-known, the U.S. Food and Drug Administration recently mandated a warning in the labels of gastric acid–suppressing medications to indicate an increase in the risk of contracting CDI.[15]

A unique and potentially modifiable exposure defined in the ICU in a single-center cohort study is *C difficile* colonization pressure (CCP).[13] CCP is defined as the sum of the daily CDI point prevalence that an individual patient is exposed to while in the unit. The incidence of CDI in this study was reported to be 3.2 per 1000 patient-days, and CCP exhibited a dose–response relationship with CDI onset, with the odds of developing CDI ranging from 0.88 for CCP greater than 0 case-days of exposure to 2.17 for CCP greater than 10 case-days. However the relationship between *C difficile* acquisition and CCP reached significance only beyond 10 case-days of exposure. And in fact, nearly one-third of all CDI cases did not experience CCP before the onset of their infection.[13] Because these data represent only a single center, where infection control measures are an emphatic part of routine care, it is difficult to know whether CCP may be a more important risk factor for ICU-acquired CDI in a setting where infection control measures are implemented with less vigor.

Marra and colleagues[16] conducted a 9-ICU single-center retrospective cohort study between 2002 and 2005 to examine the epidemiology and outcomes of CDI among patients in the ICU. Only adult patients with the first microbiologically proven CDI in the setting of diarrhea were enrolled. Among the 613 total CDI cases identified, 58 (9.5%) met the enrollment criteria. In this study, more than one-third of all incident CDI cases occurred among patients 60 years of age or older, and two-thirds were in the surgical population. More than 90% had received antibiotic before the onset of CDI, and the mean lead time to CDI development was 16.8 ± 18.5 days. Although all but one were treated with metronidazole as first-line therapy, 8.6% experienced treatment failure.[16]

Another single-center retrospective study of patients in the ICU with incident CDI reported a high proportion of elderly individuals: 53% of the 278 cases identified were 65 years of age or older.[17] The time to onset of CDI was far shorter in the older (6.4 ± 9.6 days) than in the younger (11.0 ± 19.5 days) group.[18]

OUTCOMES

A handful of studies have examined the outcomes associated with CDI in the ICU. General disagreement exists as to whether CDI is associated with an increase in mortality in this population. Thus, one single-center matched case-control study in critically ill patients calculated the death rate attributable to CDI at 6%.[17] Two other studies failed to detect an increase in mortality, however. Lawrence and colleagues[13] found no difference in hospital mortality among patients in the ICU with or without incident CDI. Similarly, Zilberberg and colleagues[12] reported essentially equal rates of unadjusted hospital death among patients on PAMV with and without CDI. In the adjusted analysis, interestingly, the discharges diagnosed with CDI seemed to have a lower risk of hospital death than those without CDI, although this was attributed to the likely presence of immortal time bias (ie, one has to remain alive to develop CDI).[12]

Several mortality predictors among patients with CDI in the ICU have been reported, the most important of which are the severity of illness and age. In the study by Marra and colleagues,[16] Sequential Organ Failure Assessment (SOFA) score and age showed a strong and independent association with hospital mortality. In another cohort focusing specifically on the elderly, high Acute Physiology and Chronic Health Evaluation II (APACHE II) score correlated strongly with hospital death.[18] Additional factors that emerged were the absence of chronic respiratory disease, age of 75 years or older, and the presence of septic shock.[18]

Although whether CDI adds to the risk of hospital mortality in patients in the ICU remains unclear, no doubt exists that it adds to hospital resource use. In the general hospitalized population, estimates show that in 2008, CDI was responsible for 2.8 to 6.4 additional days in the hospital, at a cost of $3000 to more than $15,000 per case.[11] This individual price tag adds up to between $1 billion and nearly $5 billion spent on this complication.[11] Among the critically ill, CDI is associated with a 24% increase in the risk of a longer hospitalization (95% CI, 7%–44%).[13] In the specific population of patients undergoing PAMV, CDI was associated with a 6.1-day prolongation of length of stay and additional hospital costs of $10,355.[12]

CDI PREVENTION

The principles of CDI prevention were synthesized by Cohen and colleagues[19] in the 2010 clinical practice guidelines for CDI. Pathogen transmission between patients and health care professionals is a major source of CDI infection, and therefore personal and environmental strategies are the cornerstone of combating *C difficile* proliferation. The recommendations are divided into 4 categories: (1) measures for health care workers, patients, and visitors, (2) environmental cleaning and disinfection, (3) antimicrobial use restrictions, and (4) use of probiotics. Each deserves a brief discussion.

Measures for Health Care Workers, Patients, and Visitors

The fundamental idea of this suite of interventions is to keep the infection limited to where it already exists and not allow the spores to spread to other individuals. To accomplish this, isolating all infected patients for the duration of their diarrhea symptoms is recommended. Moreover, all health care workers, even in the absence of any contact with known CDI, must follow meticulous hand hygiene protocols. Although alcohol-based hand sanitizers are deemed acceptable for use in routine practice, in the setting of an outbreak, soap and water are recommended. Recent evidence supports this recommendation, and even possibly to broaden it to routine use of soap and water. Oughton and colleagues[20] examined the efficacy of 5 different hand hygiene methods in removing *C difficile* from healthy volunteers inoculated with its spores. The groups, comprising 10 volunteers each, were exposed to (1) warm water with soap, (2) cold water with soap, (3) warm water with antibacterial soap, (4) alcohol hand wipe, and (5) alcohol hand rub. The greatest effect size for removing *C difficile* spores was detected in the warm and cold water with soap groups, followed by warm water with antibacterial soap and, finally, alcohol hand wipes. Startlingly, the average number of colony-forming units did not change at all in the alcohol hand rub group.[20] This study, albeit small, attests to the value of hand washing with soap and water as a tool to curtail the transmission of *C difficile* spores.

Gloves are another way to abrogate *C difficile* transmission. Therefore, the application of gloves on entry into a room of a patient infected with *C difficile* is recommended. Data supporting this recommendation come partly from a cluster randomized trial of intensive education regarding the use of gloves in the setting of CDI.[21] On the 2 wards randomized to the glove intervention, the incidence of CDI decreased 5-fold. At the same time, on the 2 comparable control wards with no intensive education, the CDI incidence drifted slightly lower, although not significantly.[21]

Environmental Cleaning and Disinfection

The recommendations under this rubric in the guidelines include the following 3 points: (1) environmental sources of *C difficile* should be identified and removed, including replacement of electronic rectal thermometers with disposables; (2) chlorine-containing cleaning agents or other sporicidal agents should be used to address environmental contamination; and (3) routine environmental screening for *C difficile* is not recommended.[19] Therefore, each patient in isolation should have dedicated equipment, such as stethoscopes and blood pressure cuffs, to avoid transmission to other patients through these fomites. Evidence suggests that busy health care workers do not always change their gloves after contact with contaminated commodes. In one single-center study, this behavior resulted in a 10% rate of contamination with *C difficile* spores on blood pressure cuffs, similar to the proportion of contaminated commodes (11.5%), ultimately leading to the spread of CDI.[22] Several studies have also documented reductions in CDI spread after replacement of thermometers with single-use disposable devices.[23,24]

Environmental contamination with *C difficile* is associated with disease incidence. Several strategies are available for environmental cleaning, with chlorine bleach solutions carrying the most practical benefit. A 1000 to 5000 parts per million (ppm) solution of bleach is recommeded.[19] Although the latter is more effective, the former may be more tolerable to people in and around the area. The risk/benefit balance depends on the immediacy of the CDI problem in the particular unit. Although the peroxide vaporization technique has been shown to reduce *C difficile* spores, the process does not seem practical for broad adoption. Furthermore, nonchlorine cleaners in subinhibitory concentrations seem to encourage greater sporulation of the NAP1/BI/027 strain.

Whether environmental cleaning can reduce the incidence of CDI in a nonepidemic or in low endemicity circumstances remains unclear. Mayfield and colleagues,[25] in a before-and-after study of environmental bleach disinfection, showed a sharp decrease of more than 60% in the hazard of contracting CDI on a hematopoietic stem cell transplant ward that had been experiencing high rates of this infection. The same intervention on wards that had much lower baseline incidence of CDI failed to achieve further reductions.

Antimicrobial Use Restrictions

Because the pathogenesis of CDI is closely linked to use of antimicrobial agents, it stands to reason that imprudent use of these agents leads to an increased risk of CDI. Therefore, reining in overuse of these agents is recommended to reduce the risk of *C difficile* acquisition, and data support this approach. The guidelines acknowledge this by recommending that use of all antimicrobial agents, and particularly cephalosporins and clindamycin, be reduced to the minimum number of agents and minimum duration feasible.[19] Although a Cochrane review from 2005 found conflicting results in this regard, several studies since its publication have confirmed that antimicrobial stewardship interventions are reasonable.[26] For example, in the midst of the multihospital outbreak of CDI in Quebec caused by the emerging NAP1/BI/027 strain, one of the affected hospitals reported a successful curbing of the spread of this pathogen through a nonrestrictive antibiotic control program.[27] In this instance, the antibiotic restriction effort followed on the heels of strengthened infection control measures, which failed to bring the epidemic under control. Specific antibiotic classes targeted were second- and third-generation cephalosporins, ciprofloxacin, clindamycin, and macrolides. In addition, the local guidelines suggested shortening the duration of antibiotic exposure for some specific infection types. The resulting decrease in antibiotic consumption overall, and specifically of the second- and third-generation cephalosporins, was accompanied by a significant reduction in the incidence of CDI.[27] Consistent with this role of antibiotics, a recent meta-analysis reported concomitant use of non-CDI antibiotics to be the strongest risk factor for a CDI recurrence, with an odds ratio of 4.23 (95% CI, 2.10–8.55; $P<.001$).[28]

Use of Probiotics

The Society for Healthcare Epidemiology of America/Infectious Diseases Society of America guidelines do not recommend the use of probiotics at this time.[19] This conclusion is based on several clinical trials in various settings that failed to show any advantage of probiotics compared with controls regarding CDI incidence. Although a single trial reported a reduction in CDI among patients receiving antibiotics for other infections,[29] unfortunately multiple design issues precluded these data from being generalizable to recommend this approach.

A systematic review from the Cochrane Collaboration reached the same conclusion.[30] The investigators identified only 4 studies that met their inclusion criteria, of which only one showed a benefit in reducing CDI recurrence.[31]

A more recent multicenter randomized controlled trial among patients in the ICU aimed to establish the efficacy of probiotics in preventing ventilator-associated pneumonia (VAP).[32] Specifically, the aim of this double-blind placebo-controlled randomized controlled trial was to determine whether oropharyngeal and gastric administration of *Lactobacillus rhamnosus* GG can reduce the incidence of VAP in a population of patients on mechanical ventilation at high risk for this infection. Enteral probiotics administered to 68 patients were compared with inert inulin-based placebo administered twice daily in addition to routine care among 70 controls. Microbiologically confirmed VAP occurred in 40% in the placebo group, compared with 19.1% in the *Lactobacillus* group ($P = .007$). Beyond this impact on VAP, the investigators also noted a significant reduction in CDI frequency, from 18.6% in the placebo to 5.8% in the probiotic group ($P = .02$). However, until these positive findings are incorporated into the full body of evidence on the role of probiotics in CDI prevention, whether the potential for developing invasive disease from a probiotic organism outweighs the potential benefits of these agents remains unclear.[33]

SUMMARY

C difficile is a formidable problem in the twenty-first century. Because of injudicious use of antibiotics, the emergence of the hypervirulent epidemic strain of this organism has been difficult to contain. The NAP1/BI/027 strain causes more-severe disease than other widely prevalent strains and affects patients who had not been traditionally thought to be at risk for CDI. Critically ill patients remain at high risk for this pathogen, and preventive measures, such as meticulous contact precautions, hand hygiene, environmental disinfection, and, most importantly, antibiotic stewardship, are the cornerstones of mitigation. The positive preliminary data for the role of probiotics in the ICU population are intriguing, although their risk/benefit ratio requires further confirmation.

REFERENCES

1. Pépin JL, Valiquette L, Abary ME, et al. Clostridium difficile-associated diarrhea in a region of Quebec from 1991 to 2003: a changing pattern of disease severity. CMAJ 2004;171:466–72.
2. Muto CA, Blank MK, Marsh JW, et al. Control of an outbreak of infection with the hypervirulent clostridium difficile BI strain in a university hospital using a comprehensive "bundle" approach. Clin Infect Dis 2007;45:1266–73.
3. McDonald LC, Owings M, Jernigan DB. Clostridium difficile infection in patients discharged from US short-stay hospitals, 1996–2003. Emerg Infect Dis 2006; 12:409–15.
4. Zilberberg MD, Shorr AF, Kollef MH. Increase in adult Clostridium difficile-related hospitalizations and case-fatality rate, United States, 2000–2005. Emerg Infect Dis 2008;14:929–31.
5. McDonald LC, Killgore GE, Thompson A, et al. An epidemic, toxin gene-variant strain of clostridium difficile. N Engl J Med 2005;353:2433–41.
6. Merrigan M, Venugopal A, Mallozzi M, et al. Human hypervirulent Clostridium difficile strains exhibit increased sporulation as well as robust toxin production. J Bacteriol 2010;192:4904–11.
7. Hudson M. Statistical bulletin–deaths involving clostridium difficile: England & Wales, 2009. Newport (Wales): Office for National Statistics; 2010.
8. Loo VG, Poirier L, Miller MA, et al. A predominantly clonal multi-institutional outbreak of clostridium difficile-associated diarrhea with high morbidity and mortality. N Engl J Med 2005;353:2442–9.
9. Hubert B, Loo VG, Bourgault AM, et al. A portrait of the geographic dissemination of the clostridium difficile North American pulsed-field type 1 strain and the epidemiology of C. Difficile-associated disease in Quebec. Clin Infect Dis 2007;44:238–44.
10. Chernak E, Johnson CC, Weltman A, et al. Severe clostridium difficile-associated disease in populations previously at low risk—four states, 2005. MMWR Morb Mortal Wkly Rep 2005;54:1201–5.
11. Dubberke ER, Olsen MA. Burden of Clostridium difficile on the healthcare system. Clin Infect Dis 2012;55(S2):S88–92.
12. Zilberberg MD, Nathanson BH, Sadigov S, et al. Epidemiology and outcomes of clostridium difficile-associated disease among patients on prolonged acute mechanical ventilation. Chest 2009;136:752–8.
13. Lawrence SJ, Puzniak LA, Shadel BN, et al. Clostridium difficile in the intensive care unit: epidemiology, costs, and colonization pressure. Infect Control Hosp Epidemiol 2007;28:123–30.
14. Bobo LD, Dubberke ER, Kollef MH. Clostridium difficile in the ICU: the struggle continues. Chest 2011;140:1643–53.
15. US Food and Drug Administration. FDA drug safety communication: clostridium difficile-associated diarrhea can be associated with stomach acid drugs known as proton pump inhibitors (PPIs). Available at: http://www.fda.gov/drugs/drugsafety/ucm290510.htm. Accessed October 3, 2012.

16. Marra AR, Edmond MB, Wenzel RP, et al. Hospital-acquired clostridium difficile-associated disease in the intensive care unit setting: epidemiology, clinical course and outcome. BMC Infect Dis 2007;7:42.
17. Kenneally C, Rosini JM, Skrupky LP, et al. Analysis of 30-day mortality for clostridium difficile-associated disease in the ICU setting. Chest 2007;132: 418–24.
18. Zilberberg MD, Shorr AF, Micek ST, et al. Clostridium difficile-associated disease and mortality among the elderly critically ill. Crit Care Med 2009;37: 2583–9.
19. Cohen SH, Gerding DN, Johnson S, et al. Clinical practice guidelines for clostridium difficile infection in adults: 2010 update by the Society for Healthcare Epidemiology of America (SHEA) and the Infectious Diseases Society of America (IDSA). Infect Control Hosp Epidemiol 2010;31:431–55.
20. Oughton M, Loo VG, Dendukuri N, et al. Hand hygiene with soap and water is superior to alcohol rub and antiseptic wipes for removal of clostridium difficile. Infect Control Hosp Epidemiol 2009;30(10):939–44.
21. Johnson S, Gerding DN, Olson MM, et al. Prospective, controlled study of vinyl glove use to interrupt clostridium difficile nosocomial transmission. Am J Med 1990;88:137–40.
22. Manian FA, Meyer L, Jenne J. Clostridium difficile contamination of blood pressure cuffs: a call for a closer look at gloving practices in the era of universal precautions. Infect Control Hosp Epidemiol 1996;17:180–2.
23. Brooks S, Khan A, Stoica D, et al. Reduction in vancomycin-resistant enterococcus and clostridium difficile infections following change to tympanic thermometers. Infect Control Hosp Epidemiol 1998;19:333–6.
24. Jernigan JA, Siegman-Igra Y, Guerrant RC, et al. A randomized crossover study of disposable thermometers for prevention of clostridium difficile and other nosocomial infections. Infect Control Hosp Epidemiol 1998;19:494–9.
25. Mayfield JL, Leet T, Miller J, et al. Environmental control to reduce transmission of clostridium difficile. Clin Infect Dis 2000;31:995–1000.
26. Davey P, Brown E, Fenelon L, et al. Interventions to improve antibiotic prescribing practices for hospital inpatients. Cochrane Database Syst Rev 2005;(19):CD003543.
27. Valiquette L, Cossette B, Garant M-P, et al. Impact of a reduction in the use of high-risk antibiotics on the course of an epidemic of clostridium difficile-associated disease caused by the hypervirulent NAP1/027 Strain. Clin Infect Dis 2007;45:S112–21.
28. Garey KW, Sethi S, Yadav Y, et al. Meta-analysis to assess risk factors for recurrent clostridium difficile infection. J Hosp Infect 2008;70:298–304.
29. Hickson M, D'Souza AL, Muthu N, et al. Use of probiotic lactobacillus preparation to prevent diarrhoea associated with antibiotics: randomized double blind placebo controlled trial. BMJ 2007;335:80.
30. Pillai A, Nelson R. Probiotics for treatment of clostridium difficile-associated colitis in adults. Cochrane Database Syst Rev 2008;(1):CD004611.
31. McFarland LV, Surawicz CM, Greenberg RN, et al. A randomized placebo-controlled trial of saccharomyces boulardii in combination with standard antibiotics for clostridium difficile disease. JAMA 1994;271:1913–8.
32. Morrow LE, Kollef MH, Casale TB. Probiotic prophylaxis of ventilator-associated pneumonia: a blinded, randomized, controlled trial. Am J Respir Crit Care Med 2010;182:1058–64.
33. Enache-Angoulvant A, Hennequin C. Invasive Saccharomyces infection: a comprehensive review. Clin Infect Dis 2005;41:1559–68.

Preventing Catheter-Associated Urinary Tract Infections in the Intensive Care Unit

Carol Chenoweth, MD[a,*], Sanjay Saint, MD, MPH[b]

KEYWORDS

• Prevention • Healthcare-associated • Urinary tract infection • ICU • Urinary catheter

KEY POINTS

- Catheter-associated urinary tract infection (CAUTI) is common and costly and causes substantial patient morbidity, especially in the ICU setting.
- CAUTI is often caused by hospital-based pathogens with a propensity toward antimicrobial resistance.
- Duration of urinary catheterization is the predominant risk for CAUTI; preventive measures directed at limiting placement and early removal of urinary catheters significantly improve CAUTI rates.
- Intervention bundles, collaboratives, and hospital leadership are powerful tools for implementing preventive measures for healthcare-associated infections, including CAUTI.

INTRODUCTION: MAGNITUDE OF THE PROBLEM

Healthcare-associated urinary tract infections (UTIs) account for up to 40% of infections in hospitals and 23% of infections in the intensive care unit (ICU).[1–3] The vast majority of UTIs are related to indwelling urinary catheters; approximately 70% of UTIs (and 95% of UTIs occurring in ICUs) develop in patients with urinary catheters.[4] The Centers for Disease Control and Prevention (CDC) estimated that in 2007, 139,000 CAUTIs occurred in US hospitals.

Disclosures: C.E.C.—none and S.S.—honoraria and speaking fees from academic medical centers, hospitals, specialty societies, state-based hospital associations, and nonprofit foundations (eg, Michigan Health and Hospital Association, Institute for Healthcare Improvement) for lectures about catheter-associated urinary tract infection.

[a] Division of Infectious Diseases, Departments of Internal Medicine and Infection Control and Epidemiology, University of Michigan Health System, 3119 Taubman Center, 1500 East Medical Center Drive, Ann Arbor, MI 48109-5378, USA; [b] University of Michigan Medical School, 2800 Plymouth Road, Building 16, Room 430 West, Ann Arbor, MI 48109-2800, USA

* Corresponding author.

E-mail address: cchenow@umich.edu

Crit Care Clin 29 (2013) 19–32
http://dx.doi.org/10.1016/j.ccc.2012.10.005 **criticalcare.theclinics.com**
0749-0704/13/$ – see front matter

CAUTI has significant clinical and economic consequences. Catheter-associated bacteriuria may be associated with excess mortality, even after controlling for underlying factors such as severity of illness and comorbidities; hospital-onset bloodstream infection resulting from a urinary source has a case fatality of 32.8%.[3,5] In addition, each episode of CAUTI is estimated to cost at least $600 while urinary-tract-related bloodstream infection costs at least $2,800.[6] Consequently, CAUTIs result in as much as $131 million excess direct medical costs nationwide annually.[4]

The financial implication for hospitals is underscored by the fact that since October 2008, the Centers for Medicare and Medicaid Services (CMS) no longer reimburses hospitals for the extra costs of managing a patient with hospital-acquired CAUTI.[6] Appropriately, prevention has become a priority for most hospitals, as 65% to 70% of CAUTIs are estimated to be preventable.[7] This article reviews the pathogenesis and epidemiology of CAUTI, with a focus on preventive measures for CAUTI among the critically ill.

PATHOGENESIS

Urinary catheters interfere with the normal innate defense mechanisms that prevent attachment and migration of pathogens into the bladder; these mechanisms include length of the urethra and micturition.[1,3] Biofilms, composed of clusters of microorganisms and extracellular matrix (primarily polysaccharide materials), form on both the internal lumen and external surfaces of urinary catheters.[8,9] Typically, the biofilm is composed of one type of microorganism, although polymicrobial biofilms are possible. Organisms in the biofilm grow slower than those in urine, and yet microorganisms in the biofilm may ascend the catheter in 1 to 3 days.

Microorganisms, such as *Proteus* sp, have the ability to hydrolyze urea in the biofilm and increase urinary pH. As a result, minerals may precipitate, causing mineral encrustations along the catheter or renal calculi. Biofilms are also important because they provide a protective environment from immune cells. Antimicrobials penetrate into biofilms poorly, and microorganisms grow more slowly in biofilms, decreasing the effects of many antimicrobials.[8,9]

Most microorganisms causing CAUTI enter the bladder by ascending the urethra from the perineum. Usually (66% of the time), organisms migrate in the biofilm on the external surface of the catheter. These organisms are primarily endogenous organisms colonizing the patient's intestinal tract and perineum.[10] A smaller proportion of infections (34%) are acquired from intraluminal contamination of the collection system from exogenous sources, resulting from cross-transmission of organisms from the hands of healthcare personnel.[8,10] Rarely, organisms such as *Staphylococcus aureus* cause upper UTI from hematogenous spread.

In most instances, CAUTI is caused by microorganisms from the patient's own gastrointestinal tract; however, approximately 15% of episodes of health-care-associated bacteriuria occur in clusters because of intrahospital transmission from one patient to another.[1,8] Most of these hospital-based outbreaks have been associated with improper hand hygiene of healthcare personnel.

EPIDEMIOLOGY OF CATHETER-ASSOCIATED URINARY TRACT INFECTIONS

CAUTIs make up approximately 40% of all hospital-acquired infections, but they account for a smaller proportion of healthcare-associated infections in the ICU setting. With interventions occurring across the country, rates of CAUTI in ICUs declined significantly between 1990 and 2007.[4] Rates of CAUTIs reported through the National Healthcare Safety Network (NHSN) in 2010 ranged from 4.7 infections per 1000 catheter-days in burn ICUs to 1.3 infections per 1000 catheter-days in medical/surgical ICUs.[11] CAUTIs in pediatric ICUs occur at a rate of 2.2 to 3.9 UTIs per 1000 catheter-days. General care wards have rates of CAUTI equivalent to or higher than in the ICU setting, ranging from 0.2 to 3.2 per 1000 catheter-days; the highest rates occur in rehabilitation units.[11,12]

Microbial Cause

Enterobacteriaceae are the most common pathogens associated with CAUTI, but in the ICU setting, *Candida* sp (18%), *Enterococcus* sp (10%), and *Pseudomonas aeruginosa* (9%) become more prevalent.[1,4] In addition, antimicrobial resistance in CAUTI isolates from patients in ICU has risen in recent decades. In data reported from the CDC's NHSN in 2006 to 2007, 24.8% of all *Escherichia coli* isolates from patients with CAUTIs were resistant to fluoroquinolones.[13] Many members of Enterobacteriaceae produced extended-spectrum β-lactamases; 21.2% of *Klebsiella pneumoniae* and 5.5% of *E. coli* isolates from patients with CAUTIs were resistant to ceftriaxone or ceftazidime. Even more concerning is that during this same time, 10.1% of all *K. pneumoniae* isolates from patients with CAUTIs were resistant to carbapenems.[13]

Risk Factors

Duration of catheterization is the dominant risk factor for CAUTI; up to 95% of UTIs in the ICU are associated with an indwelling urinary catheter.[4] Bacteriuria, the precursor to CAUTI, develops quickly at an average daily rate of 3% to 10% per day of catheterization. Almost 26% of patients with a catheter in place for 2 to 10 days develop bacteriuria, and virtually all patients catheterized for 1 month develop bacteriuria. Hence, catheterization for greater than 1 month is generally the definition for long-term catheterization.[1]

Box 1 outlines the major risk factors for CAUTI. Females have a higher risk of bacteriuria than males, and heavy bacterial colonization of the perineum increases this risk. Other patient factors identified in one or more studies include rapidly fatal underlying

Box 1
Risk factors associated with catheter-associated urinary tract infection

Nonmodifiable, patient-level risk factors

Female sex

Severe underlying illness

Nonsurgical disease

Age greater than 50 years

Diabetes mellitus

Serum creatinine level greater than 2 mg/dL

Modifiable risk factors

Duration of catheterization

Adherence to aseptic catheter care

Catheter insertion after the sixth day of hospitalization

Catheter insertion outside the operating room

illness, age greater than 50 years, nonsurgical disease, hospitalization in an orthopedic or urological service, catheter insertion after the sixth day of hospitalization, catheter inserted outside the operating room, diabetes mellitus, and serum creatinine level greater than 2 mg/dL at the time of catheterization. Nonadherence to aseptic catheter care recommendations have been associated with increased risk of bacteriuria, whereas systemic antimicrobial agents have a protective effect on bacteriuria (relative risk = 2.0–3.9).[1,3]

Risk factors for UTI-associated bacteremia are less clearly understood than for catheter-associated bacteriuria because catheter-associated bacteremia occurs in less than 4% of infections. Risk factors for bloodstream infections from a urinary source from early studies included infections due to *Serratia marcescens,* male sex, immunosuppressant therapy, history of malignancy, cigarette use in the past 5 years, and number of hospital-days before bacteriuria.[14,15] In a more recent study, independent risk factors for bloodstream infection included neutropenia, renal disease, and male sex.[16] These predictors for hospital-onset urinary-tract-related bloodstream infection should aid in implementing appropriate preventive practices in patients at highest risk.[16]

SURVEILLANCE FOR CATHETER-ASSOCIATED URINARY TRACT INFECTIONS

Clinical diagnosis of CAUTI remains challenging, as neither pyuria nor bacteriuria is a reliable indicator of symptomatic UTI in the setting of catheterization.[17,18] Bacteriuria in a catheterized patient is usually defined as growth of 10^2 or more colony forming units per milliliter of a predominant microorganism.[1,19] The term, bacteriuria, is often used interchangeably with UTI in the published literature, as many early studies used bacteriuria to define catheter-associated infection. However, the distinction is clinically important because asymptomatic catheter-associated bacteriuria rarely results in adverse outcomes and generally does not require treatment.[19]

Diagnosis of UTI in patients with long-term urinary catheters is particularly problematic because bacteriuria is universally present unless antimicrobial therapy is given. Fever or other systemic symptoms may be the only clinical indication of UTI, especially in patients who have spinal cord injuries.[1,3] Clinical recognition of UTI remains important because a large proportion of antimicrobials in hospitalized patients is prescribed for treatment of UTI, most often asymptomatic bacteruria.[20,21]

An essential element of any preventive program is to measure the prevalence of the condition and provide feedback of the results of interventions to the clinical care providers. The NHSN surveillance definition for healthcare-associated UTI allows for standardization and interhospital comparison of infection rates.[22] The NHSN symptomatic CAUTI rate (UTI per 1000 urinary catheter-days) is the most widely accepted measure of infection surveillance and is endorsed by the CDC, Infectious Diseases Society of America, Society for Healthcare Epidemiologists of America (IDSA-SHEA) compendium, and Association for Professionals in Infection Control and Epidemiology (APIC).[23–25] However, a population-based measure, in which 10,000 patient-days is used as the denominator, may be a better measure to assess quality improvement interventions at individual hospitals.[26]

Surveillance for CAUTI was not a priority for most hospitals earlier, perhaps due to lack of resources required to perform full hospital surveillance and the low priority given to CAUTI, as compared with other healthcare-associated infections.[27,28] Since CMS has included CAUTI as one of the hospital-acquired complications that will not be reimbursed, hospitals have renewed interest in CAUTI.[6,29] In addition, beginning in 2012, CMS has required, as a condition of participation, that hospitals submit

ICU-level CAUTI rates to NHSN. Other process or proxy measures, such as rates of asymptomatic bacteriuria, percentage of patients with indwelling catheters, percentage of catheterization with accepted indications, and duration of catheter use, have been used in studies and collaboratives with good success.[30]

PREVENTION OF CATHETER-ASSOCIATED URINARY TRACT INFECTIONS

Several guidelines exist regarding prevention of CAUTI.[23–25] General strategies are formulated for prevention of all healthcare-associated infections, whereas targeted strategies are focused at risk factors specific for CAUTI (**Box 2**).

General Strategies for Prevention

Strict adherence to hand hygiene is recommended for the prevention of all healthcare-associated infections, including UTI.[31] Most outbreaks of urinary pathogens have been linked to inadequate employee hand hygiene. The urinary tract of hospitalized patients, especially those in an ICU setting, represents a significant reservoir for multidrug-resistant organisms (MDRO). Indwelling devices, including urinary catheters, increase the risk of colonization with MDRO, and therefore, limiting their use is an important strategy for prevention of MDRO.

Reduction in use of broad-spectrum antimicrobials, as part of an overall antimicrobial stewardship program, is an important strategy to prevent development of antimicrobial resistance related to urinary catheters.[32] Repeated antimicrobial treatment of bacteriuria during long-term catheterization is a significant risk for colonization with MDRO, yet some of this use may be inappropriate.[20,21] A recent study revealed that a 1-hour educational session reduced the inappropriate use of antibiotic therapy for

Box 2
Key strategies for prevention of catheter-associated urinary tract infection

Avoid insertion of indwelling urinary catheters

- Placement only for appropriate indications (**Box 3**)
- Institutional protocols for placement, including perioperative setting.

Early removal of indwelling catheters

- Checklist or daily plan
- Nurse-based interventions
- Electronic reminders

Alternatives to indwelling catheterization

- Intermittent catheterization
- Condom catheter
- Portable bladder ultrasound scanner

Proper techniques for insertion and maintenance of catheters

- Sterile insertion
- Closed drainage system
- Avoidance of routine bladder irrigation

Consider antimicrobial catheters in some settings

Data from Refs.[23–25]

Box 3
Appropriate indications for the placement of indwelling urinary catheters

Acute anatomic or functional urinary retention or obstruction

Urinary incontinence in the setting of open perineal or sacral wounds

Perioperative use for selected surgical procedures

- Surgical procedures of anticipated long duration
- Urologic procedures
- Intraoperatively for patients with urinary incontinence
- Need for intraoperative urinary monitoring or expected large volume of intravenous infusions

Accurate monitoring of urine output

Improving comfort for end-of-life care or patient preference

From Gould CV, Umscheid CA, Agarwal RK, et al. Healthcare Infection Control Practices Advisory Committee (HICPAC). CDC guideline for prevention of catheter-associated urinary tract infections 2009. Infect Control Hosp Epidemiol 2010;31:319–26.

inpatients with urine cultures positive for MDRO.[33] In addition, audit and feedback to care providers has potential to decrease overdiagnosis of CAUTI and associated inappropriate antibiotic use.[34]

Specific Strategies for Prevention

Several guidelines have been developed or updated recently for the prevention of CAUTI.[23–25] Nevertheless, a 2005 nationwide survey identified that more than one-half of hospitals did not have a system for monitoring urinary catheters, three-quarters did not monitor duration of catheterization, and one-third did not conduct any surveillance for UTIs.[28] Surprisingly, even after enactment of the CMS nonpayment rule, in 2009, only 1 CAUTI prevention practice, use of bladder ultrasonography, was used in more than 50% of hospitals.[35] Even when focusing on ICUs, where the risk of CAUTI is highest, only a small proportion of ICUs have policies supporting bladder ultrasonography (26%), catheter removal reminders (12%), or nurse-initiated catheter discontinuation.[36] The collaborative approach to implementation of prevention measures, as detailed later, has begun to systematic changes in adoption of prevention practices.[29,37]

Limitation of use of urinary catheters

Indwelling urinary catheters are the primary risk factor for healthcare-associated UTIs, therefore, the most effective strategy for CAUTI prevention is limitation or avoidance of catheterization.[1–3] Catheter use rates vary by ICU type but range from 0.16 urinary catheter-days per patient-days in pediatric medical ICUs to 0.80 urinary catheter-days per patient-days in trauma ICUs.[11] Decreasing catheter usage may require interventions at several stages of lifecycle of a urinary catheter (**Fig. 1**).[38]

The first step toward decreasing catheter use is limiting placement of indwelling urinary catheters; catheters should be inserted only for appropriate indications (see **Box 3**). Despite these recommendations, studies indicate that urinary catheters are placed for inappropriate indications in 21% to 50% of catheterized patients.[39,40] Healthcare institutions should develop written policies and criteria for indwelling urinary catheterization based on these widely accepted indications.[24,25] Physician

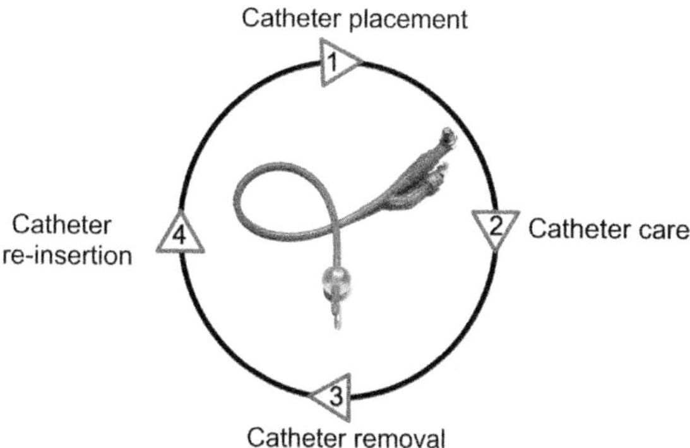

Fig. 1. Life cycle of a urinary catheter in the intensive care unit. (*From* Meddings J, Saint S. Disrupting the life cycle of the urinary catheter. Clin Infect Dis 2011;52:1291–3; with permission.)

orders should be required for insertion of any urinary catheter, and institutions should implement a system for documenting placement of catheters.[24,25]

Interventions for limiting placement of urinary catheter targeted at hospital locations where initial placement usually occurs, such as emergency departments and operating rooms, have the most impact.[41] A multifaceted approach including several types of education, system redesign, rewards, and feedback managed by a dedicated nurse resulted in a marked decrease in daily prevalence of urinary catheter-days.[42]

Once catheters are placed, strategies for early removal become essential. Urinary catheter management based on physicians' orders alone may be inadequate because physicians are frequently unaware that their patient has a urinary catheter. In one study, 28% of physicians were unaware that their patient had a catheter, with the lack of awareness increasing with the level of training.[40] In addition, physician orders for catheter placement or documentation of presence of catheter occurs in less than 50% of catheters.[43]

Nurse-driven interventions have demonstrated effectiveness in reducing duration of catheterization.[44,45] A nurse-based reminder to physicians to remove unnecessary urinary catheters in a Taiwanese hospital resulted in a reduction in CAUTI from 11.5 to 8.3 per 1000 catheter-days.[46] Such interventions are easy to implement and may consist of either a written notice or a verbal contact with the physician regarding the presence of a urinary catheter and alternative options. The feasibility of this type of intervention was demonstrated in a statewide effort that resulted in significant decrease in catheter use and increase in appropriate indications of catheters.[30]

However, computerized physician order entry systems may offer a more cost-effective and efficient system to reduce both placement of catheters and duration of catheterization. Cornia and colleagues[47] found that a computerized reminder reduced the duration of catheterization by 3 days. A systematic review and meta-analysis reports that urinary catheter reminder systems and stop orders seem to reduce the mean duration of catheterization by 37% and CAUTI by 52%.[48]

As the rate of catheterization use decreases, some centers have noted a paradoxic increase in their rate of UTI per 1000 catheter-days.[49] In reality, the actual number of CAUTIs decreased, but because of a decline in the denominator (catheter-days), the rate increased. This observation has led some experts to recommend that the rate of UTI per 10,000 patient-days be used as a more appropriate outcome measure for quality improvement interventions surrounding urinary catheters.[26]

Perioperative management of urinary catheters

Specific protocols for the management of postoperative urinary catheters are important for reducing urinary catheterization use. CMS has now included removal of urinary catheters within 24 hours of surgery as one of the Surgical Care Improvement Project (SCIP) measures that are reported by all hospitals.

Approximately, 85% of patients admitted for major surgical procedures had perioperative indwelling catheters; patients with duration of catheterization greater than 2 days were significantly more likely to develop UTIs and were less likely to be discharged home.[50] Older surgical patients were particularly at risk for prolonged catheterization; 23% of surgical patients older than 65 years were discharged to skilled nursing facilities with an indwelling catheter in place and were substantially more likely to have rehospitalization or death within 30 days.[51]

In a large prospective trial of patients undergoing orthopedic procedures, a multifaceted protocol for perioperative catheter management resulted in a two-thirds reduction in the incidence of UTI. The protocol consisted of limiting catheterization to surgeries longer than 5 hours or to total hip and knee replacements, removal of urinary catheters on postoperative day 1 after total knee arthroplasty, and postoperative day 2 after total hip arthroplasty.[52]

Evaluation of patients undergoing one of the SCIP surgeries revealed that postoperative urinary retention developed in 2.1% of patients.[53] This group has significance because it is at risk of requiring recatheterization (see **Fig. 1**). Patients who developed postoperative retention were more likely to be older men, undergoing knee, hip, or colon surgery. It will be important to focus future studies on interventions to prevent urinary retention in this higher-risk group.

Alternatives to indwelling urinary catheters

Compared with indwelling urinary catheterization, intermittent urinary catheterization reduces the risk of bacteriuria and UTI. Patients with neurogenic bladder and long-term urinary catheters, in particular, may benefit from intermittent catheterization.[24] A recent meta-analysis reported a reduced risk of asymptomatic and symptomatic bacteriuria with the use of intermittent catheterization in patients after hip or knee surgery compared with indwelling catheterization.[54] Combining the use of a portable bladder ultrasound scanner with intermittent catheterization may reduce the need for indwelling catheterization.[25,55]

Alternatively, condom catheters may be considered in place of indwelling catheters in appropriately selected male patients without urinary retention or bladder outlet obstruction. A randomized trial demonstrated a decrease in bacteriuria, symptomatic UTI, or death in patients with condom catheters, when compared with those with indwelling catheters; the benefit was primarily seen in men without dementia.[56] Condom catheters may also be less painful than indwelling catheters in some men.[56,57]

Aseptic techniques for insertion and maintenance of urinary catheters

If urinary catheterization is necessary, aseptic catheter insertion and maintenance is essential for prevention of CAUTI. Urinary catheters should be inserted by a trained healthcare professional using aseptic technique.[24,58] Cleaning the meatus before catheter insertion is recommended, but ongoing daily meatal cleaning using an antiseptic has not shown clear benefit and may increase rates of bacteriuria compared with routine care with soap and water.[1,24] Lubricant jelly should be used for insertion to reduce urethral trauma; the jelly should be sterile but antiseptic properties are not necessary.[24]

Closed urinary catheter collection systems reduce the risk of CAUTI and have been the standard of care in the United States for many years. Opening the closed system should be avoided; sampling urine may be performed aseptically from a port or from the drainage bag when large samples are required.[24,58] Prophylactic instillation of antiseptic agents or irrigation of the bladder with antimicrobial or antiseptic agents has been shown to increase infection and is not recommended.[1,24]

Reduction in bacteriuria associated with exchange of catheters is only transient, therefore routine exchange of urinary catheters is not recommended, except for mechanical reasons.[1,58] Exchange of long-term catheters at the time of treatment of symptomatic UTI, however, is likely beneficial.[59]

Use of anti-infective catheters

Antiseptic-impregnated or antimicrobial-impregnated urinary catheters have been studied extensively as an adjunctive measure for preventing CAUTI.[60–62] Antimicrobial catheters are typically coated with nitrofurazone, minocycline, or rifampin, but other agents are being evaluated in newer catheters.

In a large meta-analysis, silver alloy catheters were found to significantly reduce the incidence of asymptomatic bacteriuria in adult patients catheterized for less than 7 days, but the effect was diminished in those catheterized for greater than 7 days.[61] Similarly, antibiotic-impregnated catheters were found to decrease the rate of asymptomatic bacteriuria in those catheterized for less than 7 days but demonstrated no benefit when the duration of catheterization was greater than 7 days.[61,62] Few studies have evaluated antiseptic-coated and antibiotic-coated catheters in long-term urinary catheterization; thus, no conclusion can be drawn on use of anti-infective catheters in this setting.[63] The use of anti-infective catheters may be considered when the rates of CAUTI remain persistently high despite adherence to other evidence-based practices or in patients deemed to be at high risk for CAUTI or its complications.

Despite the fact that anti-infective urinary catheters seem to reduce bacteriuria in patients with short-term urinary catheterization, there is no convincing evidence that use of these catheters prevents CAUTI, UTI-related bloodstream infection, or mortality. Therefore, there is no recommendation for routine use of anti-infective urinary catheters to prevent CAUTI.[24] A national mixed-methods study revealed that in 2009, 45% of nonfederal and 22% of Veteran Affairs hospitals used antimicrobial catheters; hospitals using anti-infective catheters often based their decisions on hospital-specific pilot studies.[27,35]

Finally, systemic antimicrobial therapy reduces the risk of CAUTI.[1,16] However, because of issues of cost, potential adverse effects, and possible selection for

Box 4
The "ABCDE" for preventing catheter-associated urinary tract infection

- Adherence to general infection control principles (eg, hand hygiene, surveillance and feedback, aseptic insertion, proper maintenance, education) is important.
- Bladder ultrasound may avoid indwelling catheterization.
- Condom catheters or other alternatives to an indwelling catheter such as intermittent catheterization should be considered in appropriate patients.
- Do not use the indwelling catheter unless you must!
- Early removal of the catheter using a reminder or nurse-initiated removal protocol appears warranted.

From Saint S, Olmsted RN, Fakih MG, et al. Translating healthcare-associated urinary tract infection prevention research into practice via the bladder bundle. Jt Comm J Qual Patient Saf 2009;35(9):449–55; with permission.

MDRO, systemic antimicrobial therapy specifically for the purpose of preventing CAUTI is not recommended.[32]

IMPLEMENTATION: THE ROLE OF BUNDLES AND COLLABORATIVES

Recently, "bundles" of interventions have been used with resounding success for prevention of several types of healthcare-associated infections. An example of a bundle applied to CAUTI prevention is the memory aide "ABCDE" outlined in **Box 4**.[37] This bundle for preventing CAUTI was successfully adopted by the Michigan Hospital Association Keystone initiative.[30] Finally, the important role of local hospital leadership and followership for ensuring effective implementation of preventive initiatives has recently been highlighted.[64–66]

SUMMARY

CAUTIs are common, costly, and cause significant patient morbidity, especially in the ICU setting. CAUTIs are associated with hospital pathogens with a high propensity toward antimicrobial resistance. Despite studies showing benefit of interventions for prevention on CAUTI, many US healthcare facilities have not adopted these practices. Duration of urinary catheterization is the predominant risk for CAUTI; preventive measures directed at limiting placement and early removal of urinary catheters have a significant impact on decreasing CAUTI. Intervention bundles, collaboratives, and hospital leadership are powerful tools for implementation of preventive measures for healthcare-associated infections, including CAUTI.

CAUTIs account for approximately 40% of all healthcare-associated infections. As urinary catheters account for most healthcare-associated UTIs, the most important interventions are directed at avoiding placement of urinary catheters and promoting early removal when appropriate. Alternatives to indwelling catheters such as intermittent catheterization and condom catheters should be considered. If indwelling catheterization is appropriate, proper aseptic practices for catheter insertion and maintenance and a closed catheter collection system is essential for prevention of CAUTI. The use of anti-infective catheters may also be considered when the rates of CAUTI remain persistently high despite adherence to other evidence-based practices or in patients deemed to be at high risk for CAUTI or its complications. Attention toward prevention of CAUTI will likely increase because CMS and other third-party payers no longer reimburse for hospital-acquired UTIs.

REFERENCES

1. Chenoweth CE, Saint S. Urinary tract infections. Infect Dis Clin North Am 2011;25:103–17.
2. Nicolle LE. Urinary catheter-associated infections. Infect Dis Clin North Am 2012;26:13–27.
3. Shuman K, Chenoweth CE. Recognition and prevention of healthcare-associated urinary tract infections in the intensive care unit. Crit Care Med 2010;38:S373–9.
4. Burton DC, Edwards JR, Srinivasan A, et al. Trends in catheter-associated urinary tract infections in adult intensive care units-United States, 1990-2007. Infect Control Hosp Epidemiol 2011;32:748–56.
5. Chang R, Greene MT, Chenoweth CE, et al. Epidemiology of hospital-acquired urinary-tract-related bloodstream infection at a university hospital. Infect Control Hosp Epidemiol 2011;32:1127–9.

6. Saint S, Meddings JA, Calfee D, et al. Catheter-associated urinary tract infection and the Medicare rule changes. Ann Intern Med 2009;150:877–84.
7. Umsheid CA, Mitchell MD, Doshi JA, et al. Estimating the proportion of healthcare-associated infections that are reasonably preventable and the related mortality and costs. Infect Control Hosp Epidemiol 2011;32:101–14.
8. Saint S, Chenoweth CE. Biofilms and catheter-associated urinary tract infections. Infect Dis Clin North Am 2003;17:411–32.
9. Donlan RM. Biofilms and device-associated infections. Emerg Infect Dis 2001; 7(2):1–4.
10. Tambyah PA, Halvorson KT, Maki DG. A prospective study of pathogenesis of catheter-associated urinary tract infections. Mayo Clin Proc 1999;74:131–6.
11. Dudeck MA, Horan TC, Peterson KD, et al. National Healthcare Safety Network (NHSN) Report, data summary for 2010, device-associated module. Am J Infect Control 2011;39:798–816.
12. Weber DA, Sickbert-Bennett EE, Gould CV, et al. Incidence of catheter-associated urinary tract infections in a healthcare system. Infect Control Hosp Epidemiol 2011;32:822–3.
13. Hidron AI, Edwards JR, Patel J, et al. NHSN annual update: antimicrobial-resistant pathogens associated with healthcare-associated infections: annual summary of data reported to the National Healthcare Safety Network at the Centers for Disease Control and Prevention, 2006-2007. Infect Control Hosp Epidemiol 2008;29:996–1011.
14. Krieger JN, Kaiser DL, Wenzel RP. Urinary tract etiology of bloodstream infections in hospitalized patients. J Infect Dis 1983;148:57–62.
15. Saint S, Kaufman SR, Rogers MA, et al. Risk factors for nosocomial urinary tract-related bacteremia: a case-control study. Am J Infect Control 2006;34: 401–7.
16. Greene MT, Chang R, Kuhn L, et al. Predictors of hospital-acquired urinary tract-related bloodstream infection. Infect Control Hosp Epidemiol 2012;33:1001–7.
17. Musher DM, Thorsteinsson SB, Airola VM II. Quantitative urinalysis: diagnosing urinary tract infection in men. JAMA 1976;236:2069–72.
18. Tambyah PA, Maki DG. The relationship between pyuria and infection in patients with indwelling urinary catheters: a prospective study of 761 patients. Arch Intern Med 2000;160:673–7.
19. Tambyah PA, Maki DG. Catheter-associated urinary tract infection is rarely symptomatic: a prospective study of 1,497 catheterized patients. Arch Intern Med 2000;160:678–82.
20. Gandhi T, Flanders SA, Markovitz E, et al. Importance of urinary tract infection to antibiotic use among hospitalized patients. Infect Control Hosp Epidemiol 2009; 30:193–5.
21. Cope M, Cevallos ME, Cadle RM, et al. Inappropriate treatment of catheter-associated asymptomatic bacteriuria in a tertiary care hospital. Clin Infect Dis 2009;48:1182–8.
22. Centers of Disease Control and Prevention. NHSN manual: patient safety component protocols. Available at: http://www.cdc.gov/nhsn/TOC_PSCManual.html. Accessed July 23, 2012.
23. Rebmann T, Greene LR. Preventing catheter-associated urinary tract infections: an executive summary of the Association for Professionals in Infection Control and Epidemiol. Am J Infect Control 2010;38:644–6.
24. Gould CV, Umscheid CA, Agarwal RK, et al. Healthcare Infection Control Practices Advisory Committee. (HICPAC). CDC Guideline for prevention of catheter-

associated urinary tract infections 2009. Infect Control Hosp Epidemiol 2010;31: 319–26.

25. Lo E, Nicolle L, Classen D, et al. Strategies to prevent catheter-associated urinary tract infections in acute care hospitals. Infect Control Hosp Epidemiol 2008; 29(Suppl 1):S41–50.
26. Fakih MG, Greene TM, Kennedy EH, et al. Introducing a population-based outcome measure to evaluate the effect of interventions to reduce catheter-associated infection. Am J Infect Control 2012;40:359–64.
27. Saint S, Kowalski CP, Forman J, et al. A multicenter qualitative study on preventing hospital-acquired urinary tract infection in US hospitals. Infect Control Hosp Epidemiol 2008;29:333–41.
28. Saint S, Kowalski CP, Kaufman SR, et al. Preventing hospital-acquired urinary tract infection in the United States: a national study. Clin Infect Dis 2008;46:243–50.
29. Meddings J, Saint S, McMahon LF. Hospital-acquired catheter-associated urinary tract infection: documentation and coding issues may reduce financial impact of Medicare's new payment policy. Infect Control Hosp Epidemiol 2010;31:627–33.
30. Fakih MG, Watson SR, Greene T, et al. Reducing inappropriate urinary catheter use: a statewide effort. Arch Intern Med 2012;172:255–60.
31. Boyce JM, Pittet D. Guideline for hand hygiene in health-care settings. recommendations of the Healthcare Infection Control Practices Advisory Committee and the HICPAC/SHEA/APIC/IDSA hand hygiene task force. Society for Healthcare Epidemiology of America/Association for Professionals in Infection Control/ Infectious Diseases Society of America. MMWR Recomm Rep 2002;51(RR-16): 1–45.
32. Dellit TH, Owens RC, McGowan JE Jr, et al. Infectious Diseases Society of America and the Society for Healthcare Epidemiology of America guidelines for developing an institutional program to enhance antimicrobial stewardship. Clin Infect Dis 2007;44:159–77.
33. Pavese P, Saurel N, Labarere J, et al. Does an educational session with an infectious diseases physician reduce the use of inappropriate antibiotic therapy for inpatients with positive urine culture results? A controlled before-and-after study. Infect Control Hosp Epidemiol 2009;30:596–9.
34. Trautner BW, Kelly PA, Petersen N, et al. A hospital-site controlled intervention using audit and feedback to implement guidelines concerning inappropriate treatment of catheter-associated asymptomatic bacteriuria. Implement Sci 2011;6:41.
35. Krein SL, Kowalski CP, Hofer TP, et al. Preventing hospital-acquired infections: a national survey of practices reported by U.S. hospitals in 2005 and 2009. J Gen Intern Med 2012;27:773–9.
36. Conway L, Pogorzelska M, Larson E, et al. Adoption of policies to prevent catheter-associated urinary tract infections in United States intensive care units. Am J Infect Control 2012;40:705–10.
37. Saint S, Olmsted RN, Fakih MG, et al. Translating health care-associated urinary tract infection prevention research into practice via the bladder bundle. Jt Comm J Qual Patient Saf 2009;35(9):449–55.
38. Meddings J, Saint S. Disrupting the life cycle of the urinary catheter. Clin Infect Dis 2011;52:1291–3.
39. Munasinghe RL, Yazdani H, Siddique M, et al. Appropriateness of use of indwelling urinary catheters in patients admitted to the medical service. Infect Control Hosp Epidemiol 2001;22(10):647–9.
40. Saint S, Wiese J, Amory JK, et al. Are physicians aware of which of their patients have indwelling catheters? Am J Med 2000;109:476–80.

41. Fakih MG, Pena ME, Shemes S, et al. Effect of establishing guidelines on appropriate urinary catheter placement. Acad Emerg Med 2010;17:337–40.
42. Knoll BM, Wright D, Ellingson L, et al. Reduction of inappropriate urinary catheter use at a Veterans Affairs hospital through a multifaceted quality improvement project. Clin Infect Dis 2011;52:1283–90.
43. Conybeare A, Pathak S, Imam I. The quality of hospital records of urethral catheterisation. Ann R Coll Surg Engl 2002;84:109–10.
44. Fakih MG, Dueweke C, Meisner S, et al. Effect of nurse-led multidisciplinary rounds on reducing the unnecessary use of urinary catheterization in hospitalized patients. Infect Control Hosp Epidemiol 2008;29:815–9.
45. Saint S, Kaufman SR, Thompson M, et al. A reminder reduces urinary catheterization in hospitalized patients. Jt Comm J Qual Patient Saf 2005;31:455–62.
46. Huang WC, Wann SR, Lin SL, et al. Catheter-associated urinary tract infections in intensive care units can be reduced by prompting physicians to remove unnecessary catheters. Infect Control Hosp Epidemiol 2004;25:974–8.
47. Cornia PB, Amory JK, Fraser S, et al. Computer-based order entry decreases duration of indwelling urinary catheterization in hospitalized patients. Am J Med 2003;114:404–7.
48. Meddings J, Rogers MAM, Macy M, et al. Systematic review and meta-analysis: reminder systems to reduce catheter-associated urinary tract infections and urinary catheter use in hospitalized patients. Clin Infect Dis 2010; 51:550–60.
49. Wright M-O, Kharasch M, Beaumont JL, et al. Reporting catheter-associated urinary tract infections: denominator matters. Infect Control Hosp Epidemiol 2011;32:635–40.
50. Wald HL, Ma A, Bratzler DW, et al. Indwelling urinary catheter use in the postoperative period: analysis of the national surgical infection prevention project data. Arch Surg 2008;143:551–7.
51. Wald HL, Epstein AM, Radcliff TA, et al. Extended use of urinary catheters in older surgical patients: a patient safety problem? Infect Control Hosp Epidemiol 2008; 29:116–24.
52. Stephan F, Sax H, Wachsmuth M, et al. Reduction of urinary tract infection and antibiotic use after surgery: a controlled, prospective, before-after intervention study. Clin Infect Dis 2006;42:1544–51.
53. Wu AK, Auerbach AD, Aaronson DS. National incidence and outcomes of postoperative urinary retention in the surgical care improvement project. Am J Surg 2012;204:167–71.
54. Niel-Weise BS, van den Broek PJ. Urinary catheter policies for short-term bladder drainage in adults. Cochrane Database Syst Rev 2005;(3):CD004203.
55. Stevens E. Bladder ultrasound: avoiding unnecessary catheterizations. Medsurg Nurs 2005;14:249–53.
56. Saint S, Kaufman SR, Rogers MA, et al. Condom versus indwelling urinary catheters: a randomized trial. J Am Geriatr Soc 2006;54:1055–61.
57. Saint S, Lipsky BA, Baker PD, et al. Urinary catheters: what type do men and their nurses prefer? J Am Geriatr Soc 1999;47:1453–7.
58. Pratt RJ, Pellowe C, Loveday HP, et al. Guidelines for preventing infections associated with the insertion and management of short term indwelling urethral catheters in acute care. J Hosp Infect 2001;47(Suppl):S39–46.
59. Raz R, Schiller D, Nicolle LE. Chronic indwelling catheter replacement before antimicrobial therapy for symptomatic urinary tract infection. J Urol 2000;164: 1254–8.

60. Stensballe J, Tvede M, Looms D, et al. Infection risk with nitrofurazone-impregnated urinary catheters in trauma patients: a randomized trial. Ann Intern Med 2007;147:285–93.
61. Schumm K, Lam T. Types of urethral catheters for management of short-term voiding problems in hospitalised adults. Cochrane Database Syst Rev 2008;(2): CD004013.
62. Johnson JR, Kuskowski MA, Wilt TJ. Systematic review: antimicrobial urinary catheters to prevent catheter-associated urinary tract infection in hospitalized patients. Ann Intern Med 2006;144:116–26.
63. Jahn P, Preuss M, Kernig A, et al. Types of indwelling urinary catheters for long-term bladder drainage in adults. Cochrane Database Syst Rev 2007;(3):CD004997.
64. Saint S, Kowalski CP, Banaszak-Holl J, et al. The importance of leadership in preventing healthcare-associated infection: results of a multistate qualitative study. Infect Control Hosp Epidemiol 2010;31:901–7.
65. Saint S, Kowalski CP, Banaszak-Holl J, et al. How active resisters and organizational constipators affect health-care-acquired infection prevention efforts. Jt Comm J Qual Patient Saf 2009;35:239–46.
66. Damschroder LJ, Banaszak-Holl J, Kowalski CP, et al. The role of the champion in infection prevention: results from a multisite qualitative study. Qual Saf Health Care 2009;18:434–40.

Ventilator-associated Complications, Including Infection-related Complications

The Way Forward

Marin H. Kollef, MD

KEYWORDS

• VAP • VAC • Pneumonia • ICU

KEY POINTS

- Optimizing the care of mechanically ventilated patients is an important goal for health care providers and hospital administrators.
- An easily acquired and reliable marker of medical quality has been elusive for this patient population.
- Ventilator-associated complications (VACs) represent a potential solution to this problem. VACs can be easily monitored for and obtained, being defined by changes in oxygenation and/or positive end-expiratory pressure.
- The potential also exists to track VACs automatically using hospital informatics systems.
- It is important to first establish that VACs are preventable, and not simply markers of disease severity, to use them as true markers of medical quality for purposes of interinstitutional comparison and reimbursement.

INTRODUCTION

Ventilator-associated pneumonia (VAP) is one of the most common infections occurring in mechanically ventilated patients requiring antibiotic administration. Because VAP has historically been associated with excess morbidity and mortality in critically ill patients, it has been used as an overall marker of the quality of care associated with mechanical ventilation. Although recent studies have challenged the association between VAP and increased mortality, there is greater consensus that VAP is associated with prolonged durations of mechanical ventilation, increased intensive care unit (ICU) length of stay, and increased hospital costs.[1–4] Bekaert and colleagues[5]

This work was supported by the Barnes-Jewish Hospital Foundation.
Washington University School of Medicine, 660 South Euclid Avenue, St Louis, MO 63110, USA
E-mail address: mkollef@dom.wustl.edu

Crit Care Clin 29 (2013) 33–50
http://dx.doi.org/10.1016/j.ccc.2012.10.004 criticalcare.theclinics.com

estimated that 4.4% of the deaths in the ICU on day 30 and 5.9% on day 60 are attributable to VAP. As opposed to previous studies, these investigators simultaneously accounted for the time of acquiring VAP, loss to follow-up after ICU discharge, and the existence of complex feedback relations between VAP and disease severity. Kollef and colleagues[4] showed, in a matched cohort, that patients with VAP had longer mean durations of mechanical ventilation (21.8 vs 10.3 days), ICU stay (20.5 vs 11.6 days), hospitalization (32.6 vs 19.5 days), and costs ($99,598 vs $59,770) than patients without VAP.

One of the major clinical issues related to the management of mechanically ventilated patients in the ICU is the increasing occurrence of infections, including VAP, caused by multidrug-resistant (MDR) or extremely drug-resistant (XDR) pathogens.[6] The available evidence suggests that the overall prevalence of nosocomial infections attributed to MDR and XDR pathogens, as well as the global use of antibiotics in the hospital setting, is not diminishing despite local and national efforts to curb these infections.[7,8] Disorders such as tracheobronchitis and sepsis, which often are diagnosed in the presence of nosocomial pneumonia, seem to be more common, contributing, at least in part, to the increasing use of antibiotics in the ICU.[9] VAP is recognized to be among the most common infections associated with MDR and XDR bacteria including *Pseudomonas aeruginosa*, *Acinetobacter* species, and *Klebsiella pneumonia* carbapenemase–containing Enterobacteriaceae.[8–19] The recent recognition of Enterobacteriaceae containing the NDM1 gene in multiple continents raises the possibility of endemic spread of common enteric bacteria possessing resistance to all currently available antibacterial agents.[11]

The major concern related to the emergence of MDR and XDR pathogens as a cause of VAP is the inability to empirically treat these infections when they are initially suspected. Inappropriate initial antimicrobial therapy, defined as an antimicrobial regimen that lacks in vitro activity against the isolated organism(s) responsible for the infection, has been associated with excess mortality in patients with serious infections, including VAP and severe sepsis.[10,16,20–23] This is largely related to increasing bacterial resistance to antibiotics as a result of their greater use and the limited availability of newer agents.[6,17] Escalating rates of antimicrobial resistance lead many clinicians to empirically treat critically ill patients with presumed infection with a combination of broad-spectrum antibiotics, which can further perpetuate the cycle of increasing resistance.[17] Inappropriate initial antimicrobial therapy can, conversely, lead to treatment failures and adverse patient outcomes.[18,22] Moreover, the limited diversity of available antimicrobial agents has created a clinical situation in which patients are repetitively exposed to the same class of antibiotic, or, in some circumstances, the same agent, resulting in an increased risk of treatment failure and mortality.[19] Therefore, the broader concern for all intensivists is how to limit the emergence and spread of MDR/XDR pathogens, as well as the infections associated with these pathogens.

A recent international point prevalence ICU study found the lungs to be the most common site of infection, accounting for 64% of infections, followed by the abdomen (20%), the bloodstream (15%), and the renal tract/genitourinary system (14%).[9] Despite important geographic variations, *Enterococcus faecium*, *Staphylococcus aureus*, *K pneumoniae*, *Acinetobacter baumannii*, *P aeruginosa*, and *Enterobacter* species (ESKAPE) pathogens constitute more than 80% of VAP episodes.[9,15] Their clinical importance relies on their virulence and ability to develop mechanisms conferring decreased susceptibility to antimicrobials, increasing inappropriate therapy and negatively affecting the outcomes of patients in the ICU. These studies highlight the overall importance of pulmonary infections as a major cause of morbidity and antibiotic use in the ICU. However, given concerns about current diagnostic criteria for VAP, especially for assessing the clinical impact of infection prevention or quality-improvement programs on patient outcomes, other indicators of ICU care quality have been explored.[24,25]

PROBLEMATIC DEFINITION OF VAP

Clinical criteria are known to be nonspecific for the diagnosis of nosocomial pneumonia, including VAP. Clinical findings such as fever, leukocytosis, and purulent secretions occur with other noninfectious pulmonary conditions such as atelectasis, pulmonary contusion, and acute respiratory distress syndrome (ARDS), and therefore lack specificity for the diagnosis of VAP.[26–29] Chest radiographs can similarly be nonspecific for the diagnosis of nosocomial pneumonia. Wunderink and colleagues[30] found that no roentgenographic sign correlated well with the presence of pneumonia in mechanically ventilated patients. The presence of air bronchograms was the only roentgenographic sign that correlated with autopsy-verified pneumonia, correctly predicting 64% of cases. The most frequently used clinical diagnosis of VAP has traditionally required the presence of a new or progressive consolidation on chest radiology plus at least 2 of the following clinical criteria: fever greater than 38°C, leukocytosis or leukopenia, and purulent secretions. This definition has been supported by several medical specialty groups,[31,32] despite the lack of specificity of these criteria.[27–30]

The Centers for Disease Control and Prevention (CDC)/National Healthcare Safety Network (NHSN) has established a clinical definition for the presence of probable nosocomial pneumonia including VAP.[33] However, these diagnostic criteria have not been validated and at least 1 study found that decision making using these criteria was not accurate, potentially resulting in the withholding of antibiotics in 16% of patients diagnosed with VAP by bronchoalveolar lavage (BAL).[34] We recently compared the observed rates of VAP when using the CDC/NHSN surveillance method versus the American College of Chest Physicians (ACCP) clinical criteria.[35] Over 1 year, 2060 patients required mechanical ventilation for greater than 24 hours and were prospectively evaluated. Of these, 83 patients (4%) had VAP according to the ACCP criteria, compared with 12 patients (0.6%) using the CDC/NHSN surveillance method. The corresponding rates of VAP were 8.5 versus 1.2 cases per 1000 ventilator days, respectively. Agreement of the 2 sets of criteria was poor (κ statistic, 0.26). Quantitative lower respiratory tract cultures were positive in 88% of patients in the ACCP group and 92% in the NHSN group.[35]

Others have noted that surveillance rates of VAP are decreasing, whereas clinical diagnoses of VAP and tracheobronchitis, as well as antibiotic prescribing, remain prevalent.[36] External reporting pressures may be encouraging stricter interpretation of subjective signs that can cause an artifactual lowering of VAP rates. The result is that it is almost impossible to disentangle the relative contribution of quality-improvement efforts in the ICU versus surveillance effects as explanations for the currently observed low VAP rates.[36] Given the limitations of clinical criteria for establishing the diagnosis of VAP, alternative methods have been pursued. Torres and colleagues[37] used quantitative cultures of respiratory specimens obtained by BAL, protected BAL (pBAL), protected specimen brush, and tracheobronchial aspirate (TBA), which were compared with histology of lung biopsy samples to establish the diagnosis of VAP. Sensitivities for the diagnosis of VAP ranged from 16% to 37% when only histologic reference tests were used, whereas specificity ranged from 50% to 77%. When lung histology of guided or blind specimens and microbiology of lung tissue were combined, all quantitative diagnostic techniques achieved higher, but still limited, diagnostic yields (sensitivity 43%–83%; specificity 67%–91%).[37]

Similar diagnostic accuracy has been shown by other investigators using histologic criteria as a reference standard, suggesting that quantitative cultures of lower respiratory secretions may be of limited value.[27,38–45]

To simplify the technical requirements for establishing a microbiologic diagnosis of VAP, Riaz and colleagues[46] compared nonquantitative and quantitative respiratory secretion cultures for the diagnosis of VAP. These investigators found that nonquantitative culture of BAL was good at ruling out the presence of VAP but was poor at establishing the presence of VAP because of the low specificity of the test. Despite the limited overall accuracy of quantitative lower respiratory tract cultures for the diagnosis of VAP, the clinical use of such cultures has been associated with less overall antibiotic use,[47–50] which presumably results from clinicians having greater confidence in ruling out VAP with negative quantitative culture results. Similar reductions in the duration of antibiotic therapy prescribed for clinically suspected VAP have been shown using serum procalcitonin thresholds, Clinical Pulmonary Infection Score (CPIS) values, and targeted protocols.[51–54]

Given that VAP surveillance is time consuming, potentially less accurate than clinical/microbiologic criteria,[34,35] and the use of quantitative lower respiratory tract cultures for the establishment of VAP is not universally performed, the CDC Epicenters Program (CDC-PEP) has recently supported efforts to shift ICU surveillance away from VAP. Instead, the CDC-PEP has focused on the occurrence of complications in general that might circumvent the VAP definition's subjectivity and inaccuracy, facilitate electronic assessment, make interfacility comparisons more meaningful, and encourage broader prevention strategies. Ventilator-associated complications (VACs) was selected as a more general marker and was defined by sustained increases in patients' ventilator settings after a period of stable or decreasing support (**Box 1**).

The use of VAC as an outcome predictor was examined in a recent CDC-PEP study of 597 mechanically ventilated patients.[55] These investigators found that 9.3% of their study population developed VAP (8.8 per 1000 ventilator days) whereas 23% had a VAC (21.2 per 1000 ventilator days). Compared with matched controls, both VAP and VAC prolonged days to extubation (5.8, 95% confidence interval [CI] 4.2–8.0 and 6.0, 95% CI 5.1–7.1 respectively), days to ICU discharge (5.7, 95% CI 4.2–7.7 and 5.0, 95% CI 4.1–5.9), and days to hospital discharge (4.7, 95% CI 2.6–7.5 and 3.0, 95% CI 2.1–4.0). VAC was associated with increased mortality (odds ratio [OR] 2.0, 95% CI 1.3–3.2) but VAP was not (OR 1.1, 95% CI 0.5–2.4). VAC assessment was also faster (mean 1.8 minutes vs 39 minutes per patient). Both VAP and VAC events were predominantly attributable to pneumonia, pulmonary edema, ARDS, and atelectasis. The investigators concluded that screening for VAC captures a similar set of complications to traditional VAP surveillance but is faster, more objective, and potentially a superior predictor of clinical outcomes.

Building on their experience with VAC, the CDC-PEP has begun to evaluate a new streamlined surveillance definition for VAP (sVAP) (**Table 1**) based on their experience with VAC. The same investigators retrospectively compared surveillance time, reproducibility, and outcomes for streamlined versus conventional surveillance definitions of VAP among medical and surgical patients on mechanical ventilation in 3 university hospitals.[56] Application of the streamlined definition was faster (mean 3.5 minutes vs 39.0 minutes per patient) and more objective than the conventional definition. On multivariate analysis, the streamlined definition predicted increases in ventilator days, intensive care days, and hospital mortality as effectively as conventional surveillance. Although sVAP does not necessarily reflect the presence of bacterial pneumonia, it is hoped that this marker will allow quality-improvement efforts to be more accurately assessed across time periods and institutions compared with the traditional use of VAP as a quality indicator.[57] However, neither VAC or sVAP have been evaluated in terms of potentially modifying antibiotic consumption or reducing the emergence of antibiotic-resistant bacteria in the ICU setting.

An accompanying editorial from the CDC-PEC suggested that the NHSN is committed to completing and implementing new quality criteria for critically ill patients in the form of VAC and IVAC (see **Box 1**).[58] These streamlined quality criteria will undergo a period of review from various critical care groups and societies (Society of Critical Care Medicine, American Association of Respiratory Care, ACCP, American Thoracic Society, and American Society of Critical Care Nurses) before their expected acceptance and implementation by the National Quality Forum and the Centers for Medicare & Medicaid Services. With input from these key constituents, NHSN is prepared to make changes that will maximize reliable case identification, be responsive to new scientific findings, and simplify implementation through use of advances in health information technology, while maintaining clinical and epidemiologic credibility through partnerships with key providers and state health departments. The hope is that implementation of these new surveillance criteria will allow the quality of medical care to be more accurately assessed in the ICU setting. However, to accomplish these goals, most VACs and IVACs have to be shown to be preventable to effectively link them to health care quality.

BUNDLES FOR QUALITY IMPROVEMENT AND THE PREVENTION OF VAP

More than a decade ago, an education-based program at Barnes-Jewish Hospital directed toward respiratory care practitioners and ICU nurses was developed by a multidisciplinary task force to highlight correct practices for the prevention of VAP.[59] Each participant was required to take a preintervention test before reviewing a study module and an identical postintervention test after completion of the study module. Following implementation of the education module, the rate of VAP decreased to 5.7 per 1000 ventilator days from 12.6 per 1000 ventilator days.[59] The cost savings secondary to the decreased rate of VAP for the 12 months following the intervention was estimated to be greater than $400,000. This educational protocol was then implemented across the 4 largest hospitals in the local health care system.[60] VAP rates for all 4 hospitals combined decreased by 46%, from 8.75/1000 ventilator days in the year before the intervention to 4.74/1000 ventilator days in the 18 months following the intervention ($P<.001$). Statistically significant decreased rates were observed at the pediatric hospital and at 2 of the 3 adult hospitals. No significant change in VAP rates was seen at the community hospital with the lowest rate of study module completion among respiratory therapists (56%). In addition to showing the effectiveness of a bundle for VAP prevention, these studies highlight the importance of compliance with the elements of the bundle to ensure its success. This same education-based bundle package has also been successfully used in the ICUs of a hospital in Thailand.[61]

Lansford and colleagues[62] also developed a simple bundle for the prevention of VAP in patients with trauma, focusing on head of bed elevation, oral cleansing with chlorhexidine, a once-daily respiratory therapist–driven weaning attempt, and conversion of nasogastric to orogastric feeding tubes. Implementation of this bundle was associated with a significant reduction in the rate of VAP. Elements of this bundle have also been shown to be effective in other surgical/trauma units at Barnes-Jewish Hospital.[63] However, compliance with infection control protocols often wanes over time and can be significantly influenced by staffing levels in the ICU.[64] Some

Box 1
Criteria for VACs, infection-related VACs (IVACs), possible VAP, and probable VAP proposed by the CDC-PEP[a]

VAC

Patient has a baseline period of stability or improvement on the ventilator, defined by 2 or more calendar days of stable or decreasing Fio_2 or PEEP. Baseline Fio_2 and PEEP are defined by the minimum daily Fio_2 or PEEP measurement during the period of stability or improvement.

After a period of stability or improvement on the ventilator, the patient has at least 1 of the following indicators of worsening oxygenation:

1. Minimum daily Fio_2 values increase greater than or equal to 0.20 (20 points) more than baseline and remain equal to or more than that increased level for 2 or more calendar days
2. Minimum daily PEEP values increase greater than or equal to 3 cm H_2O more than baseline and remain equal to or more than that increased level for 2 or more calendar days

IVAC

On or after calendar day 3 of mechanical ventilation and within 2 calendar days before or after the onset of worsening oxygenation, the patient meets both of the following criteria:

1. Temperature greater than 38°C or less than 36°C, or white blood cell count greater than or equal to 12,000 cells/mm^3 or less than or equal to 4000 cells/mm^3
2. A new antimicrobial agent(s) is started, and is continued for greater than or equal to 4 calendar days

Possible VAP

On or after calendar day 3 of mechanical ventilation and within 2 calendar days before or after the onset of worsening oxygenation, 1 of the following criteria is met:

1. Purulent respiratory secretions (from 1 or more specimen collections)
   a. Defined as secretions from the lungs, bronchi, or trachea that contain more than 25 neutrophils and less than 10 squamous epithelial cells per low-power field
   b. If the laboratory reports semiquantitative results, those results must be equivalent to the quantitative thresholds presented earlier
2. Positive culture (qualitative, semiquantitative, or quantitative) of sputum, endotracheal aspirate, BAL, lung tissue, or protected specimen brushing

Probable VAP

On or after calendar day 3 of mechanical ventilation and within 2 calendar days before or after the onset of worsening oxygenation, 1 of the following criteria is met:

1. Purulent respiratory secretions (from 1 or more specimen collections and defined as for possible VAP)

And 1 of the following:

   a. Positive culture of endotracheal aspirate, greater than or equal to 10^5 CFU/mL, or equivalent semiquantitative result
   b. Positive culture of BAL, greater than or equal to 10^4 CFU/mL, or equivalent semiquantitative result
   c. Positive culture of lung tissue, greater than or equal to 10^4 CFU/mL, or equivalent semiquantitative result
   d. Positive culture of protected specimen brush, greater than or equal to 10^3 CFU/mL, or equivalent semiquantitative result

2. One of the following (without requirement for purulent respiratory secretions):
   a. Positive pleural fluid culture (specimen obtained during thoracentesis or initial placement of chest tube and not from an indwelling chest tube)
   b. Positive lung histopathology
   c. Positive diagnostic test for *Legionella* spp
   d. Positive diagnostic test on respiratory secretions for influenza virus, respiratory syncytial virus, adenovirus, parainfluenza virus

Abbreviations: CFU, colony-forming units; Fio_2, fraction of inspired oxygen; PEEP, positive end-expiratory pressure.
[a] Note that only VAC and IVAC are intended for public reporting.

institutions have used computerized flow sheets and quality rounding checklists in the ICU to improve compliance with care measures involved in the prevention of VAP, as well as other complications (eg, deep vein thrombosis, stress ulcer formation).[65–67] Berenholtz and colleagues[68] implemented a statewide multifaceted intervention to improve compliance with 5 evidence-based recommendations for mechanically ventilated patients and to prevent VAP. One-hundred and twelve ICUs reporting 3228 ICU months and 550,800 ventilator days showed the VAP rate to have decreased from a mean of 6.9 cases per 1000 ventilator days at baseline to a mean of 3.4 cases per 1000 ventilator days at 16 to 18 months after implementation.[68]

Rello and colleagues[69] conducted a VAP prevention study in 5 Spanish adult ICUs focusing on 5 evidence-based measures (avoidance of ventilator circuit changes unless clinically indicated, use of sedation control protocols, strict hand hygiene, oral care with chlorhexidine, intracuff pressure control of the endotracheal tube). Despite modest compliance with these interventions that varied between 16.4% (oral care) and 34.0% (no circuit changes), the prevention intervention achieved reductions in VAP rates, ICU length of stay, and duration of mechanical ventilation.

Bouadma and colleagues[70] published their experience with a multimodal comprehensive intervention strategy for VAP prevention with a strong emphasis on process control. This French intervention included a multidisciplinary task force, an educational session, direct observations with performance feedback, technical improvements, and scheduled reminders. Eight evidence-based bundled interventions were systematically rolled out and used, including hand hygiene, preferably alcohol-based hand-rubbing; glove and gown use for endotracheal tube manipulation; backrest elevation of 30° to 45°; tracheal cuff pressure maintenance greater than 20 cm H_2O; use of orogastric tubes; avoidance of gastric overdistension; oral hygiene with chlorhexidine; and elimination of nonessential tracheal suction. The investigators carefully monitored compliance with process indicators and VAP rates over the study period. Compliance assessment consisted of five 4-week periods (before the intervention and at 1, 6, 12, and 24 months thereafter). Compliance with procedures such as hand hygiene or wearing gloves and gowns for endotracheal tube handling were already high at study entry and remained so. Other procedures such as backrest elevation or correct tracheal cuff pressure maintenance were low and did not increase until the introduction of 2 prompts. Overall quality improvement, measured by a continuous increase in compliance with the 8 prevention measures, resulted in a 51% reduction of VAP rates.[70]

Bouadma and colleagues focused on process control rather than outcome measure for sustained practice improvement and benchmarking, which is a compelling

Table 1
Comparison of conventional and streamlined surveillance definitions for VAP

	Conventional Definition	Streamlined Definition
Radiology	Two or more serial chest radiographs with at least 1 of the following: 1. New or progressive and persistent infiltrate 2. Consolidation 3. Cavitation	Two or more serial chest radiographs with at least 1 of the following: 1. New or progressive and persistent infiltrate 2. Consolidation 3. Cavitation
Systemic signs (at least 1)	1. Fever (>38°C or >100.4°F)	1. Fever (>38°C or >100.4°F)
	2. Leukopenia (<4000 WBC/mm^3) or leukocytosis (≥12 000 WBC/mm^3)	2. Leukopenia (<4000 WBC/mm^3) or leukocytosis (≥12 000 WBC/mm^3)
	3. For adults ≥70 years old, altered mental status with no other recognized cause	—
Pulmonary signs (at least 2)	1. New onset of purulent sputum, or change in character of sputum, or increased respiratory secretions, or increased suctioning requirements	1. ≥25 neutrophils per low-power field on Gram stain of endotracheal aspirate or bronchoalveolar lavage specimen
	2. Worsening gas exchange (eg, desaturations, increased oxygen requirements, or increased ventilator demand)	2. ≥2 days of stable or decreasing daily minimum PEEP followed by an increase in daily minimum PEEP of ≥2.5 cm H_2O, sustained for ≥2 calendar days; or ≥2 days of stable or decreasing daily minimum Fio_2 followed by an increase in daily minimum Fio_2 of ≥0.15 points, sustained for ≥2 calendar days
	3. New-onset or worsening cough, or dyspnea, or tachypnea	—
	4. Rales or bronchial breath sounds	—

Abbreviation: WBC, white blood cell.

approach in the light of the unsettled dilemma of VAP definitions and the impact of case mix.[71] The main advantage of such an approach is the objectivity of the process elements, which can more accurately be quantified than VAP. In addition, these same investigators compared VAP rates during a 45-month baseline period and a 30-month intervention period in a cohort of patients who received mechanical ventilation for greater than 48 hours.[72] Baseline and intervention VAP rates were 22.6 and 13.1 total VAP episodes over total mechanical ventilation duration per 1000 ventilation-days, respectively (*P*<.001). These cumulative data support the use of targeted approaches for the reduction of VAP despite the limitations of the criteria used for defining VAP. They also highlight the importance of VAP as a quality indicator despite the abovementioned limitations. It will be crucial to conduct similar studies using VAC or IVAC as the quality end point to determine whether similar benefits in outcomes can be achieved.

SELECTING PROCESS ELEMENTS TO INCLUDE IN VAP PREVENTION BUNDLES

The Institute for Healthcare Improvement (IHI) has put forward the simplest ventilator bundle, consisting of 4 evidence-based practices to improve the outcomes of mechanical ventilation: (1) peptic ulcer disease prophylaxis, (2) deep venous thrombosis prophylaxis, (3) elevation of head of the bed, and (4) daily sedation vacation and assessment of readiness to wean.[73] Only 2 of these bundle elements (elevation of the head of the bed and sedation vacations) have been specifically evaluated as VAP prevention measures. Despite methodological flaws, a recent systematic review identified 4 peer-reviewed studies that assessed in various degrees the effect of implementing the IHI ventilator bundle on the incidence of VAP.[74] In these studies, the incidence of VAP decreased from the range of 2.7 to 13.3 cases to 0.0 to 9.3 cases per 1000 ventilator days. In addition, 2 of the 4 studies noted a directional decline in the average ICU length of stay. The IHI bundle approach to VAP prevention, although attractively simple on the surface, may represent only an incremental first, and seemingly sensible, step to translating evidence into practice, the impact of which nevertheless remains unknown. The investigators of this review also concluded that the IHI VAP bundle and other seemingly sensible approaches to VAP prevention need to be examined for their clinical effectiveness and cost-effectiveness, particularly because new technologies or prevention strategies coming to market will require evaluation of their comparative effectiveness.[75–77]

Other investigations have used more targeted elements in their bundles specifically aimed at the prevention of VAP.[59–61] As previously noted, Bouadma and colleagues[70] implemented a rigorous bundle with 8 evidence-based elements directly linked to the prevention of VAP. More recently, Heimes and colleagues[78] performed a retrospective study examining 696 consecutive ventilated patients in a level 1 trauma center to evaluate a VAP prevention bundle with 7 elements (elevate head of bed 30° or higher unless contraindicated; twice-daily oral cleansing with chlorhexidine; daily respiratory therapy–driven attempt to liberate from mechanical ventilation; nasogastric tubes replaced with orogastric tubes; sedation held and monitored daily to allow patients to follow commands; stress gastritis prophylaxis with H_2 blockers or proton pump inhibitors; hand washing by health care personnel). Three time periods were assessed: pre-VAP bundle implementation, VAP bundle implementation, and a subsequent time period of VAP bundle enforcement. During the pre-VAP bundle period, 5.2 cases of VAP occurred per 1000 days of ventilator support compared with 2.4/1000 days ($P = .172$) and 1.2/1000 days ($P = .085$) in the implementation and enforcement periods, respectively. However, when all trauma patients were included, regardless of head Abbreviated Injury Score (AIS) score, the difference in the rate of VAP was statistically significant in the enforcement period, but not in the implementation period, compared with the pre-VAP bundle period ($P = .014$ and .062, respectively). In contrast with the study by Rello and colleagues,[60,69,70] this study supports the need for strict enforcement or compliance with VAP bundles to maximize their successful implementation.

One of the main advantages of bundled approaches for the prevention of VAP is their simplicity and, as a result, their cost-effectiveness. VAP prevention programs have been successfully implemented in developing countries with limited resource expenditures.[61,79] The implementation of VAP preventive measures grouped into bundles is a strategy that has consistently been shown to improve effectiveness, because the combined use of interventions is expected to achieve better outcomes than when interventions are implemented individually.[80–83] The measures that compose a bundle should be chosen based on the available scientific evidence and the expected resource availability at the local hospital level. Even when compliance with the bundle is not fully achieved, a reduction in the incidence of VAP is possible.[69,82] Similar bundles intended to prevent VACs or IVACs should be validated in prospective studies.

Box 2
SMART approach to quality control

Specific quality-improvement interventions

- Use evidence-based bundle elements
- Ensure that local resources are capable of supporting selected bundle elements
- Do not become bound to any single bundle element if it is ineffective or impractical to implement

Measurable outcome

- Focus on compliance with process elements
- Select limited but clinically relevant outcome measures (eg, VAP incidence, antibiotic use, duration of mechanical ventilation)
- Guard against reporting biases, especially when using before-after or time-series methods

Achievable program

- Target 1 problem or outcome at a time
- Do not overreach local resource capability
- Develop a local approach to quality improvement that can be applied to subsequent problems or outcomes

Relevant quality-improvement program

- Target problems or outcomes that have direct clinical significance and consequences to patient care (eg, improved compliance with sedation holiday protocols or infection control protocols)
- Update quality-improvement programs as new information, technology, or resources become available
- Use periodic reviews of all quality-improvement programs by unbiased individuals to evaluate their success and cost-effectiveness

Time-bound program

- Use discrete time periods for the implementation and evaluation of each quality-improvement program
- Develop objective parameters to determine whether quality-improvement interventions should continue, be modified, or be discontinued
- Avoid having quality-improvement programs in place without definite periods of reevaluation

SPECIFIC, MEASURABLE, ACHIEVABLE, RELEVANT, TIME-BOUND APPROACHES FOR QUALITY IMPROVEMENT AND THE PREVENTION OF COMPLICATIONS IN THE ICU

Evidence-based interventions are available to reduce the occurrence of VAP, especially when these interventions are bundled together.[59–61,70] To increase the likelihood of success, clinicians and administrators should follow a specific, measurable, achievable, relevant, time-bound (SMART) approach for the implementation of such quality-improvement efforts (**Box 2**, **Fig. 1**).[84] Process-improvement initiatives in the hospital should choose specific objectives that precisely define and quantify desired outcomes, such as reducing the rate of VAP by 25% or improving compliance with specific processes (eg, compliance with identifiable VAP prevention interventions to a predetermined goal level). Such efforts should avoid unrealistic objectives, such as attempting to completely eliminate VAP or VACs, which could result in biased underreporting of VAP, or other complications, to meet the desired goal. A practical process improvement should be implemented in a way that allows both measurement of the outcome (VAP, VAC, IVAC, sVAP) and staff adherence to the elements making up the bundle for the process-improvement project. All objectives should be achievable and relevant by engaging stakeholders and empowering them to select specific tactics and steps for implementation. Nurses, respiratory therapists, and other stakeholders are in the best position to identify the preventive tactics that are achievable within their busy ICUs. Begin with simple, cost-effective tactics. Anticipate the need to add more tactics or bundle elements to achieve the desired process implementation and targeted infection/complication rates, and consider the use of certain measures designed to enforce the use of the prevention or quality-improvement program (**Box 3**).

All process-improvement efforts should be periodically reviewed to assess compliance with their elements and sustained ability to achieve targeted goals, and to introduce advances in technology or behavioral science techniques. Bouadma and colleagues[70,72] showed the ability of such rigorous methods to produce sustained VAP rate decreases in the long term. However, these investigators also showed that VAP rates remained substantial at their institution despite high compliance with

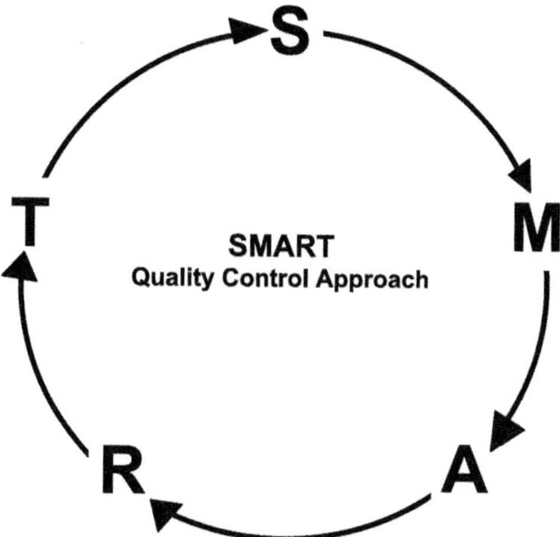

Fig. 1. A SMART program for process improvement and quality control.

Box 3
Bundle elements for a mechanical ventilation quality program

Mandatory elements

- Strict hand disinfection before patient contacts
- Use of noninvasive mask ventilation when possible
- Orotracheal intubation preferred (when tracheal intubation is necessary)
- Orogastric intubation preferred for gastric access
- Appropriate use of analgesia and sedation (daily spontaneous awakening trials when stable)
- Daily spontaneous breathing trials (in conjunction with daily spontaneous awakening trials)
- Use of checklists or computerized order sets to optimize bundle compliance
- Adequate ICU staffing
- Avoidance of unplanned extubations and reintubations
- Deep vein thrombosis prophylaxis
- Gastrointestinal bleeding prophylaxis
- Semierect positioning unless contraindicated because of hemodynamics (eg, shock) or therapeutics (extracorporeal membrane oxygenation)
- Avoid ventilator circuit changes unless clinically indicated
- Early use of physical therapy and mobilization

Other elements for bundle consideration

- Avoidance of patient transports unless clearly clinically indicated
- Use of closed endotracheal suctioning
- Subglottic secretion drainage
- Adequate endotracheal tube cuff pressure
- Oral chlorhexidine
- Appropriate nutritional support (to include optimal delivery route)
- Glucose control
- Pressure sore avoidance strategy in place

Enforcement measures

- Computerized order sets for bundle elements
- Use of rounding checklists
- Compliance assessments using random surveillance or observation periods
- Distribution of report cards and infection rates
- Involvement of hospital leadership in the review of prevention program outcomes
- Scheduled in-services, educational briefings, and town hall sessions to review procedures, outcomes, and barriers to successful bundle implementation

preventive measures, suggesting that elimination of VAP, or other VACs, may be an unrealistic goal. Therefore, the focus of such quality-improvement efforts should be process driven to maximize the benefits of available hospital resources for the desired goal (eg, reduced occurrence of VAP or VACs).

SUMMARY

Given the rising costs of health care and limited government budgets, process improvement, safety, and quality should be hardwired into the culture of hospitals, and this is becoming increasingly evident as more institutions are adopting Toyota-inspired quality management strategies to improve quality as well as to reduce hospital costs.[85] Moreover, until more objective surveillance end points, such as sVAP, VAC, or IVAC, are developed and validated, it will be difficult to compare quality-improvement efforts across sites or to know what levels of improved medical care (eg, zero VAP or VAC rates) can be achieved.

Health care providers and hospital administration should strive to provide the highest level of medical care possible. Nowhere is this more important than high-intensity resource areas such as the ICU. Intensivists, critical care nurses, and other support personnel will continue to be challenged to keep pace with rapidly advancing changes in medical care and technology. The use of a simplified quality indicator, such as VAC or IVAC, holds the promise of allowing quality to be surveyed over time and across centers. However, it is imperative that such markers of quality first be validated as representing preventable events that can be intervened on.

REFERENCES

1. Nguile-Makao M, Zahar JR, Francais A, et al. Attributable mortality of ventilator-associated pneumonia: respective impact of main characteristics at ICU admission and VAP onset using conditional logistic regression and multi-state models. Intensive Care Med 2010;36:781–9.
2. Shorr AF, Zilberberg MD, Kollef M. Cost-effectiveness analysis of a silver-coated endotracheal tube to reduce the incidence of ventilator-associated pneumonia. Infect Control Hosp Epidemiol 2009;30:759–63.
3. Warren DK, Shukla SJ, Olsen MA, et al. Outcome and attributable cost of ventilator-associated pneumonia among intensive care unit patients in a suburban medical center. Crit Care Med 2003;31:1312–7.
4. Kollef MH, Hamilton CW, Ernst FR. Economic impact of ventilator-associated pneumonia in a large matched cohort. Infect Control Hosp Epidemiol 2012;33: 250–6.
5. Bekaert M, Timsit JF, Vansteelandt S, et al. Attributable mortality of ventilator-associated pneumonia: a reappraisal using causal analysis. Am J Respir Crit Care Med 2011;184:1133–9.
6. Arias CA, Murray BE. Antibiotic-resistant bugs in the 21st century–a clinical super-challenge. N Engl J Med 2009;360:439–43.
7. Chung R, Song J-H, Kim SH, et al. High prevalence of multidrug-resistant non-fermenters in hospital-acquired pneumonia in Asia. Am J Respir Crit Care Med 2011;184:1409–17.
8. Kallen AJ, Hidron AI, Patel J, et al. Multidrug resistance among gram-negative pathogens that caused healthcare-associated infections reported to the National Healthcare Safety Network, 2006-2008. Infect Control Hosp Epidemiol 2010;31: 528–31.
9. Vincent JL, Rello J, Marshall J, et al. International study of the prevalence and outcomes of infection in intensive care units. JAMA 2009;302:2323–9.
10. Kollef KE, Schramm GE, Wills AR, et al. Predictors of 30-day mortality and hospital costs in patients with ventilator-associated pneumonia attributed to potentially antibiotic-resistant gram-negative bacteria. Chest 2008;134:281–7.

11. Centers for Disease Control and Prevention (CDC). Detection of Enterobacteriaceae isolates carrying metallo-beta-lactamase - United States, 2010. MMWR Morb Mortal Wkly Rep 2010;59:750.
12. Cantón R, Akóva M, Carmeli Y, et al. Rapid evolution and spread of carbapenemases among *Enterobacteriaceae* in Europe. Clin Microbiol Infect 2012;18: 413–31.
13. Viau RA, Hujer AM, Marshall SH, et al. "Silent" Dissemination of *Klebsiella pneumoniae* isolates bearing *K. pneumoniae* carbapenemase in a long-term care facility for children and young adults in northeast Ohio. Clin Infect Dis 2012;54: 1314–21.
14. Lee YT, Kuo SC, Yang SP, et al. Impact of appropriate antimicrobial therapy on mortality associated with *Acinetobacter baumannii* bacteremia: relation to severity of infection. Clin Infect Dis 2012;55(2):209–15.
15. Sandiumenge A, Rello J. Ventilator-associated pneumonia caused by ESKAPE organisms: cause, clinical features, and management. Curr Opin Pulm Med 2012;18:187–93.
16. Ferrer R, Artigas A, Suarez D, et al. Effectiveness of treatments for severe sepsis: a prospective, multicenter, observational study. Am J Respir Crit Care Med 2009; 180:861–6.
17. Boucher H, Talbot GH, Bradley JS, et al. Bad bugs, no drugs: no ESKAPE! An update from the Infectious Diseases Society of America. Clin Infect Dis 2009; 48:1–12.
18. Kollef MH. Broad-spectrum antimicrobials and the treatment of serious bacterial infections: getting it right up front. Clin Infect Dis 2008;47:S3–13.
19. Johnson MT, Reichley R, Hoppe-Bauer J, et al. Impact of previous antibiotic therapy on outcome of Gram-negative severe sepsis. Crit Care Med 2011;39: 1859–65.
20. Kollef MH, Sherman G, Ward S, et al. Inadequate antimicrobial treatment of infections: a risk factor for hospital mortality among critically ill patients. Chest 1999; 115:462–74.
21. Dhainaut JF, Laterre PF, LaRosa SP, et al. The clinical evaluation committee in a large multicenter phase 3 trial of drotrecogin alfa (activated) in patients with severe sepsis (PROWESS): role, methodology, and results. Crit Care Med 2003;31:2291–301.
22. Garnacho-Montero J, Garcia-Garmendia JL, Barrero-Almodovar A, et al. Impact of adequate empirical antibiotic therapy on the outcome of patients admitted to the intensive care unit with sepsis. Crit Care Med 2003;31:2742–51.
23. Harbarth S, Garbino J, Pugin J, et al. Inappropriate initial antimicrobial therapy and its effect on survival in a clinical trial of immunomodulating therapy for severe sepsis. Am J Med 2003;115:529–35.
24. Halpern NA, Hale KE, Sepkowitz KA, et al. A world without ventilator-associated pneumonia: time to abandon surveillance and deconstruct the bundle. Crit Care Med 2012;40:267–70.
25. Kollef MH. Prevention of ventilator-associated pneumonia or ventilator-associated complications: a worthy, yet challenging, goal. Crit Care Med 2012;40:271–7.
26. Morrow LE, Kollef MH. Recognition and prevention of nosocomial pneumonia in the intensive care unit and infection control in mechanical ventilation. Crit Care Med 2010;38:S352–62.
27. Tejerina E, Esteban A, Fernandez-Segoviano P, et al. Accuracy of clinical definitions of ventilator-associated pneumonia: comparison of autopsy findings. J Crit Care 2010;25:62–6.

28. Rea-Neto A, Youssef NC, Tuche F, et al. Diagnosis of ventilator-associated pneumonia: a systematic review of the literature. Crit Care 2008;12:R56.
29. Vincent JL, de Souza Barros D, Cianferoni S. Diagnosis, management, and prevention of ventilator-associated pneumonia. Drugs 2010;70:1927–44.
30. Wunderink RG, Woldenberg LS, Zeiss J, et al. The radiologic diagnosis of autopsy-proven ventilator-associated pneumonia. Chest 1992;101:458–63.
31. Pingleton SK, Fagon JY, Leeper KV Jr. Patient selection for clinical investigation of ventilator-associated pneumonia. Criteria for evaluating diagnostic techniques. Chest 1992;102:553S–6S.
32. American Thoracic Society; Infectious Diseases Society of America. Guidelines for the management of adults with hospital-acquired, ventilator-associated, and healthcare-associated pneumonia. Am J Respir Crit Care Med 2005;71:388–416.
33. Centers for Disease Control and Prevention: National Nosocomial Infections Surveillance System (NNIS). Available at: http://www.cdc.gov/ncidod/dhqp/nnis.html. Accessed March 7, 2012.
34. Miller PR, Johnson JC, Karchmer T, et al. National nosocomial infection surveillance system: from benchmark to bedside in trauma patients. J Trauma 2006;60:98–103.
35. Skrupky L, McConnell K, Dallas J, et al. A comparison of ventilator-associated pneumonia rates as identified according to National Healthcare Safety Network (NHSN) and American College of Chest Physicians (ACCP) Criteria. Crit Care Med 2012;40:281–4.
36. Klompas M. Is a ventilator-associated pneumonia rate of zero really possible? Curr Opin Infect Dis 2012;25:176–82.
37. Torres A, Fabregas N, Ewig S, et al. Sampling methods for ventilator-associated pneumonia: validation using different histologic and microbiological references. Crit Care Med 2000;28:2799–804.
38. Balthazar AB, Von NA, De Capitani EM, et al. Diagnostic investigation of ventilator-associated pneumonia using bronchoalveolar lavage: comparative study with a postmortem lung biopsy. Braz J Med Biol Res 2001;34:993–1001.
39. Torres A, el-Ebiary M, Padró L, et al. Validation of different techniques for the diagnosis of ventilator-associated pneumonia. Comparison with immediate postmortem pulmonary biopsy. Am J Respir Crit Care Med 1994;149:324–31.
40. Torres A, El-Ebiary M, Fábregas N, et al. Value of intracellular bacteria detection in the diagnosis of ventilator associated pneumonia. Thorax 1996;51:378–84.
41. Kirtland SH, Corley DE, Winterbauer RH, et al. The diagnosis of ventilator-associated pneumonia: a comparison of histologic, microbiologic, and clinical criteria. Chest 1997;112:445–57.
42. Marquette CH, Copin MC, Wallet F, et al. Diagnostic tests for pneumonia in ventilated patients: prospective evaluation of diagnostic accuracy using histology as a diagnostic gold standard. Am J Respir Crit Care Med 1995;151:1878–88.
43. Papazian L, Autillo-Touati A, Thomas P, et al. Diagnosis of ventilator-associated pneumonia: an evaluation of direct examination and presence of intracellular organisms. Anesthesiology 1997;87:268–76.
44. Rouby JJ, Rossignon MD, Nicolas MH, et al. A prospective study of protected bronchoalveolar lavage in the diagnosis of nosocomial pneumonia. Anesthesiology 1989;71:679–85.

45. Fàbregas N, Ewig S, Torres A, et al. Clinical diagnosis of ventilator associated pneumonia revisited: comparative validation using immediate post-mortem lung biopsies. Thorax 1999;54:867–73.
46. Riaz OJ, Malhotra AK, Aboutanos MB, et al. Bronchoalveolar lavage in the diagnosis of ventilator-associated pneumonia: to quantitate or not, that is the question. Am Surg 2011;77:297–303.
47. Fagon JY, Chastre J, Wolff M, et al. Invasive and noninvasive strategies for management of suspected ventilator-associated pneumonia. A randomized trial. Ann Intern Med 2000;132:621–30.
48. Shorr AF, Sherner JH, Jackson WL, et al. Invasive approaches to the diagnosis of ventilator-associated pneumonia: a meta-analysis. Crit Care Med 2005;33:46–53.
49. Ibrahim EH, Ward S, Sherman G, et al. Experience with a clinical guideline for the treatment of ventilator-associated pneumonia. Crit Care Med 2001;29:1109–15.
50. Dellit TH, Chan JD, Skerrett SJ, et al. Development of a guideline for the management of ventilator-associated pneumonia based on local microbiologic findings and impact of the guideline on antimicrobial use practices. Infect Control Hosp Epidemiol 2008;29:525–33.
51. Bouadma L, Luyt CE, Tubach F, et al. Use of procalcitonin to reduce patients' exposure to antibiotics in intensive care units (PRORATA trial): a multicentre randomised controlled trial. Lancet 2010;375:463–74.
52. Stolz D, Smyrnios N, Eggimann P, et al. Procalcitonin for reduced antibiotic exposure in ventilator-associated pneumonia: a randomised study. Eur Respir J 2009; 34:1364–75.
53. Micek ST, Ward S, Fraser VJ, et al. A randomized controlled trial of an antibiotic discontinuation policy for clinically suspected ventilator-associated pneumonia. Chest 2004;125:1791–9.
54. Singh N, Rogers P, Atwood CW, et al. Short-course empiric antibiotic therapy for patients with pulmonary infiltrates in the intensive care unit. A proposed solution for indiscriminate antibiotic prescription. Am J Respir Crit Care Med 2000;162:505–11.
55. Klompas M, Khan Y, Kleinman K, et al. Multicenter evaluation of a novel surveillance paradigm for complications of mechanical ventilation. PLoS One 2011;6: e18062.
56. Klompas M, Kleinman K, Khan Y, et al. Rapid and reproducible surveillance for ventilator-associated pneumonia. Clin Infect Dis 2012;54:370–7.
57. Uçkay I, Ahmed QA, Sax H, et al. Ventilator-associated pneumonia as a quality indicator for patient safety? Clin Infect Dis 2008;46:557–63.
58. Magill SS, Fridkin SK. Improving surveillance definitions for ventilator-associated pneumonia in an era of public reporting and performance measurement. Clin Infect Dis 2012;54:378–80.
59. Zack JE, Garrison T, Trovillion E, et al. Effect of an education program aimed at reducing the occurrence of ventilator-associated pneumonia. Crit Care Med 2002;30:2407–12.
60. Babcock HM, Zack JE, Garrison T, et al. An educational intervention to reduce ventilator-associated pneumonia in an integrated health system. A comparison of effects. Chest 2004;125:2224–31.
61. Apisarnthanarak A, Pinitchai U, Thongphubeth K, et al. Effectiveness of an educational program to reduce ventilator-associated pneumonia in a tertiary care center in Thailand: a 4-year study. Clin Infect Dis 2007;45:704–11.
62. Lansford T, Moncure M, Carlton E, et al. Efficacy of a pneumonia prevention protocol in the reduction of ventilator-associated pneumonia in trauma patients. Surg Infect (Larchmt) 2007;8:505–10.

63. Sona CS, Zack JE, Schallom ME, et al. The impact of a simple, low-cost oral care protocol on ventilator-associated pneumonia rates in a surgical intensive care unit. J Intensive Care Med 2009;24:54–62.
64. Kollef MH. Prevention of hospital-associated pneumonia and ventilator-associated pneumonia. Crit Care Med 2004;32:1396–405.
65. DuBose JJ, Inaba K, Shiflett A, et al. Measurable outcomes of quality improvement in the trauma intensive care unit: the impact of a daily quality rounding checklist. J Trauma 2008;64:22–7.
66. Wahl WL, Talsma A, Dawson C, et al. Use of computerized ICU documentation to capture ICU core measures. Surgery 2006;140:684–9.
67. Weiss CH, Moazed F, McEvoy CA, et al. Prompting physicians to address a daily checklist and process of care and clinical outcomes: a single-site study. Am J Respir Crit Care Med 2011;184:680–6.
68. Berenholtz SM, Pham JC, Thompson DA, et al. Collaborative cohort study of an intervention to reduce ventilator-associated pneumonia in the intensive care unit. Infect Control Hosp Epidemiol 2011;32:305–14.
69. Rello J, Afonso E, Lisboa T, et al. A care bundle approach for prevention of ventilator-associated pneumonia. Clin Microbiol Infect 2012. [Epub ahead of print].
70. Bouadma L, Mourvillier B, Deiler V, et al. A multifaceted program to prevent ventilator-associated pneumonia: impact on compliance with preventive measures. Crit Care Med 2010;38:789–96.
71. Pittet D, Zingg W. Reducing ventilator-associated pneumonia: when process control allows outcome improvement and even benchmarking. Crit Care Med 2010;38:983–4.
72. Bouadma L, Deslandes E, Lolom I, et al. Long-term impact of a multifaceted prevention program on ventilator-associated pneumonia in a medical intensive care unit. Clin Infect Dis 2010;51:1115–22.
73. Institute for healthcare improvement. Available at: http://www.ihi.org. Accessed June 3, 2011.
74. Zilberberg MD, Shorr AF, Kollef MH. Implementing quality improvements in the intensive care unit: ventilator bundle as an example. Crit Care Med 2009;37:305–9.
75. Kollef MH, Afessa B, Anzueto A, et al. Silver-coated endotracheal tubes and incidence of ventilator-associated pneumonia: the NASCENT randomized trial. JAMA 2008;20(300):805–13.
76. Lorente L, Blot S, Rello J, et al. New issues and controversies in the prevention of ventilator-associated pneumonia. Am J Respir Crit Care Med 2010;182:870–6.
77. Muscedere J, Rewa O, McKechnie K, et al. Subglottic secretion drainage for the prevention of ventilator-associated pneumonia: a systematic review and meta-analysis. Crit Care Med 2011;39:1985–91.
78. Heimes J, Braxton C, Nazir N, et al. Implementation and enforcement of ventilator-associated pneumonia prevention strategies in trauma patients. Surg Infect (Larchmt) 2011;12:99–103.
79. Rosenthal VD, Alvarez-Moreno C, Villamil-Gómez W, et al. Effectiveness of a multidimensional approach to reduce ventilator-associated pneumonia in pediatric intensive care units of 5 developing countries: International Nosocomial Infection Control Consortium findings. Am J Infect Control 2011;40(6):497–501.
80. Al-Tawfiq JA, Abed MS. Decreasing ventilator-associated pneumonia in adult intensive care units using the Institute for Healthcare Improvement bundle. Am J Infect Control 2010;38:552–6.

81. Morris AC, Hay AW, Swann DG, et al. Reducing ventilator-associated pneumonia in intensive care: impact of implementing a care bundle. Crit Care Med 2011;39: 2218–24.
82. Ramirez P, Bassi GL, Torres A. Measures to prevent nosocomial infections during mechanical ventilation. Curr Opin Crit Care 2012;18:86–92.
83. Rewa O, Muscedere J. Ventilator-associated pneumonia: update on etiology, prevention, and management. Curr Infect Dis Rep 2011;13:287–95.
84. Kollef M. SMART approaches for reducing nosocomial infections in the ICU. Chest 2008;134:447–56.
85. Culig MH, Kunkle RF, Frndak DC, et al. Improving patient care in cardiac surgery using Toyota production system based methodology. Ann Thorac Surg 2011;91: 394–9.

Preventing Delirium in the Intensive Care Unit

Nathan E. Brummel, MD[a,b,c,*], Timothy D. Girard, MD, MSCI[a,b,c,d]

KEYWORDS

• Delirium • Intensive care unit • Prevention • Sedation

KEY POINTS

- Delirium in the intensive care unit (ICU) is exceedingly common, and risk factors for delirium among the critically ill are nearly ubiquitous.
- Addressing modifiable risk factors including sedation management, deliriogenic medications, immobility, and sleep disruption can help to prevent and reduce the duration of this deadly syndrome.
- The ABCDE approach to critical care is a bundled approach that clinicians can implement for many patients treated in their ICUs to prevent the adverse outcomes associated with delirium and critical illness.

INTRODUCTION

Delirium in the intensive care unit (ICU) represents an acute form of organ dysfunction, which manifests as a rapidly developing disturbance of both consciousness and cognition that tends to fluctuate throughout the course of a day.[1] The American Psychiatric Association (APA) *Diagnostic and Statistical Manual of Mental Disorders*, fourth edition, text revision (DSM-IV) defines 4 key features of delirium: (1) disturbance of consciousness with reduced awareness of the environment and impaired ability to focus, sustain, or shift attention; (2) altered cognition (eg, impaired memory, language disturbance, or disorientation) or the development of a perceptual disturbance (eg,

Funding source: NIH (Grant numbers: K23AG034257; T32HL087738).
The authors have no financial conflicts to disclose.

[a] Division of Allergy, Pulmonary, and Critical Care Medicine, Department of Medicine, Vanderbilt University School of Medicine, Nashville, TN 37232, USA; [b] Department of Medicine, Center for Health Services Research, Vanderbilt University School of Medicine, Nashville, TN 37232, USA; [c] Geriatric Research, Education and Clinical Center (GRECC) Service, Department of Veterans Affairs Medical Center, Tennessee Valley Healthcare System, 1310 24th Avenue South, Nashville, TN 37212, USA; [d] Department of Medicine, Center for Quality of Aging, Vanderbilt University School of Medicine, Nashville, TN 37232, USA

* Corresponding author. Medical Center East, 6th Floor, 1215 21st Avenue South, Suite 6000, Nashville, TN 37232.
E-mail address: nathan.brummel@vanderbilt.edu

Crit Care Clin 29 (2013) 51–65
http://dx.doi.org/10.1016/j.ccc.2012.10.007 criticalcare.theclinics.com
0749-0704/13/$ – see front matter

hallucinations, delusions, or illusions) that is not better accounted for by preexisting or evolving dementia; (3) disturbance that develops over a short period of time (hours to days) and tends to fluctuate during the course of the day; and (4) evidence of an etiologic factor (ie, delirium due to general medical condition, substance-induced delirium, delirium due to multiple causes, or delirium not otherwise specified).[1]

Delirium is common in the ICU, affecting 60% to 80% of mechanically ventilated patients and 20% to 50% of nonmechanically ventilated patients.[2–8] Its presence heralds both short-term and long-term adverse outcomes. In the hospital, delirious patients are at increased risk for prolonged mechanical ventilation, catheter removal, self-extubation, and the need for physical restraints.[3,9,10] In addition, delirium predisposes patients to longer hospital stays, with greater health care costs, increased risk of death during the hospitalization, and increased odds of institutionalization following discharge.[10–15] Even after hospital discharge, the amount of time a patient has been delirious in the ICU predicts long-term cognitive impairment, physical disability, and death up to a year later.[12,16–20]

Given the common occurrence of delirium and the adverse outcomes associated with its presence, preventing delirium in the ICU is a key factor in enhancing the quality of care in ICUs worldwide. However, before considering preventive strategies one must first ask whether delirium in the ICU can be prevented from developing in the first place. Although some ICU patients develop delirium from a single, preventable risk factor—and thus, recognition and avoidance or minimization of this risk factor may effectively prevent the patient from developing delirium—delirium more often occurs when a vulnerable patient (ie, having multiple predisposing risk factors) encounters a large insult or insults (ie, develops a precipitating risk factor).[21] Frequently the insult causing delirium is the critical illness leading to ICU admission, such that a large number of patients are delirious before arrival in the ICU. Indeed, delirium commonly occurs in conjunction with other acute organ failures such as respiratory failure, shock, and/or renal failure. By the time of ICU admission, the "horse is out of the barn" for many patients, because the syndrome has already developed and therefore cannot be prevented. Even in these patients, however, "preventive" strategies may be of benefit through their effect on the duration of delirium. Multiple studies have found that the number of days an ICU patient is delirious is associated with numerous adverse outcomes, including cognitive impairment, physical disability, and death in the year following a critical illness.

This article reviews strategies to prevent not only the development of delirium in critically ill patients but also to prevent the persistence of delirium in the ICU, which may be a more attainable goal. Many of these strategies are part of the recently described ABCDE approach to ICU care, which clinicians can use to address modifiable risk factors associated with delirium and to improve outcomes for their patients.

RISK FACTORS FOR DELIRIUM

The average medical ICU patient has 11 or more risk factors for developing delirium,[11] which can be divided into baseline (predisposing) and hospital-related (precipitating) factors.[21] Baseline risk factors are those relating to a patient's underlying characteristics and comorbidities, and hospital-related factors are those relating to the patient's acute illness, its treatment, and ICU management (**Table 1**). These risk factors combine to cause delirium in a given patient such that a highly vulnerable patient may develop delirium with only a minor insult (eg, an elderly patient with underlying dementia may develop delirium from a simple urinary tract infection), whereas a less vulnerable patient often requires a greater insult or insults to develop delirium

Table 1
Risk factors for delirium

	Unmodifiable/Unpreventable Risk Factors	Potentially Modifiable/ Preventable Risk Factors
Baseline risk factors	Age APOE-4 genotype History of hypertension Preexisting cognitive impairment History of alcohol use History of tobacco use History of depression	Sensory deprivation (ie, hearing or vision impairment)
Acute illness–related risk factors	High severity of illness Respiratory disease Medical illness (vs surgical) Need for mechanical ventilation Number of infusing medications Elevated inflammatory biomarkers High LNAA metabolite levels	Anemia Acidosis Hypotension Infection/sepsis Metabolic disturbances (eg, hypocalcemia, hyponatremia, azotemia, transaminitis, hyperamylasemia, hyperbilirubinemia) Fever
Hospital-related risk factors	Lack of daylight Isolation	Lack of visitors Sedatives/analgesics (eg, benzodiazepines and opiates) Immobility Bladder catheters Vascular catheters Gastric tubes Sleep depravation

Critically ill patients are exposed to a multitude of risk factors for delirium relating to baseline comorbidities, acute illness, and treatment in the hospital/ICU. These risk factors may be viewed as unmodifiable/unpreventable or potentially modifiable/preventable. Delirium prevention in the ICU should focus on reducing the number and duration of potentially modifiable/preventable risk factors.

Abbreviations: APOE-4, apolipoprotien-E4 polymorphism; CRP, C-reactive protein; LNAA, large neutral amino acids.

(eg, a younger patient without predisposing risk factors who develops delirium in the setting of septic shock and acute respiratory distress syndrome requiring mechanical ventilation). In general, risk factors relating to the patient's acute illness and its treatment are potentially more modifiable than baseline risk factors; altering these risk factors may thus serve as one means to prevent delirium in the ICU.

DELIRIUM PREVENTION IN NON-ICU PATIENTS

Multicomponent strategies to prevent the development of delirium have yet to be fully developed and studied in the ICU, but an overview of strategies for delirium prevention that have been examined carefully in other populations in which delirium is prevalent, namely hospitalized elderly patients and those undergoing hip-fracture repair (**Fig. 1**), is likely informative for ICU clinicians despite the current paucity of evidence in this setting. Inouye and colleagues,[22] for example, studied a protocol aimed at reducing common risk factors for delirium among acutely ill elderly patients. The protocol targeted sleep deprivation, disorientation, immobility, dehydration, and visual and hearing

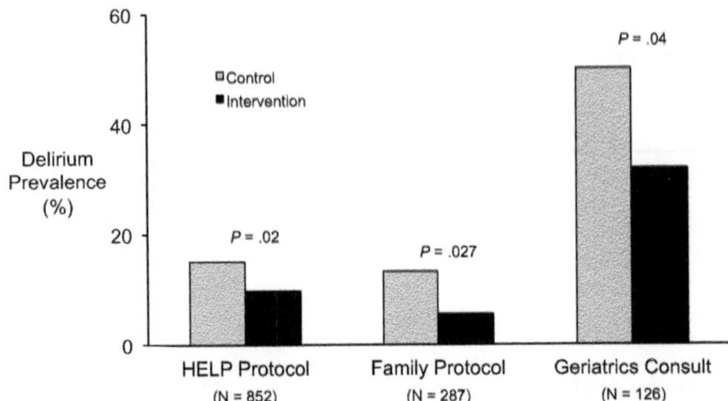

Fig. 1. Prevalence of delirium in nonpharmacologic delirium prevention trials. Inouye and colleagues[22] studied the Hospital Elder Life Program (HELP) protocol in hospitalized elderly, and found a reduction in delirium prevalence from 15% among patients in the usual care group to 9.9% among patients in the intervention group. A similar protocol, studied by Martinez and colleagues,[23] used family members to deliver the nonpharmacologic interventions to acutely ill elderly patients, and found a reduction in delirium prevalence from 13.3% in the usual care group to 5.6% in the intervention group. Marcantonio and colleagues[24] found that a geriatrics consultation in patients undergoing surgical fixation of hip fractures reduced delirium from 50% in patients not receiving a consultation to 32% in patients who received a consultation.

impairment. In a randomized controlled trial, this multifaceted intervention was associated with a 40% relative reduction in the development of delirium in the intervention group. Of note, this intervention was more effective at preventing delirium than treating it once it had developed. In another randomized trial, the efficacy of a delirium prevention protocol delivered by patients' family members was established. Family members were taught to recognize the signs and symptoms of delirium, to reorient their loved ones by providing them with familiar objects such as family pictures, and to provide eyeglasses and hearing aids to avoid of sensory deprivation. These interventions reduced the number of cases of incident delirium by half.[23] A third randomized trial explored the effect of an early geriatrics consultation on the development of delirium among patients undergoing surgical hip-fracture repair.[24] The geriatricians took a protocolized approach to reducing the number of potentially deliriogenic medications, provided adequate analgesic medications, controlled blood pressure, prevented hypoxemia, and ensured the presence of eyeglasses and hearing aids. These interventions resulted in an 18% absolute reduction in incident delirium during the study period. In summary, all 3 of these well-designed, randomized trials demonstrated that nonpharmacologic interventions targeting multiple risk factors can reduce the prevalence of delirium in susceptible populations of non–critically ill patients.

Other trials examined whether pharmacologic interventions, namely prophylactic antipsychotics, can prevent delirium in postoperative populations; these trials yielded mixed results. Elderly hip-surgery patients, for example, who were randomized to haloperidol prophylaxis (rather than placebo) beginning before surgery and continuing for up to 3 days postoperatively, did not experience any reduction in the incidence of postoperative delirium. The haloperidol group did, however, have significantly shorter duration of delirium and a shorter hospital stay, suggesting that interventions intended to prevent delirium may be beneficial despite the occurrence of delirium.[25] A second trial in patients undergoing joint arthroplasty compared olanzapine with placebo, and did find a significantly lower incidence of postoperative delirium in the olanzapine group.[26] In another trial, elective cardiac surgery patients randomized to risperidone immediately following surgery were less likely than those randomized to placebo to develop postoperative delirium compared with placebo.[27] These trials suggest that prophylactic administration of antipsychotics may reduce the incidence of delirium in certain populations at high risk for developing delirium.

Of importance, the overall incidence of delirium in these non-ICU populations is much lower than those observed in the ICU, where patients are typically exposed to many more risk factors than those affecting non-ICU patients. Thus, the overall effectiveness of these preventive interventions may not be generalizable to the ICU, and further investigation of these strategies in the critically ill is needed. Nevertheless, nonpharmacologic interventions targeting specific modifiable risk factors such as removing catheters when no longer needed, providing reorientation to confused patients, and ensuring the availability of eyeglasses and hearing aids are low-risk, low-cost approaches that may be easily implemented in the ICU and therefore warrant consideration as prevention strategies in the ICU. Prophylactic antipsychotic administration has been studied in small ICU cohorts, and this is discussed later in this article.

DELIRIUM PREVENTION IN ICU PATIENTS

On the whole, the constellation of risk factors for delirium affecting individual ICU patients varies from patient to patient and thus an individualized strategy for delirium prevention should be sought. Nonetheless, 3 risk factors in particular, sedatives, immobility, and sleep disruption, are widespread in the ICU as a result of clinical practice habits in most ICUs and therefore serve as important targets for delirium prevention. In addition, antipsychotics and cholinesterase inhibitors intended to prevent delirium in the ICU have been studied, although the results to date have not suggested that their use is warranted.

Preventing Delirium Through Management of Sedatives

The use of sedatives is nearly ubiquitous among patients receiving mechanical ventilation in the ICU.[28] A complete description of best practices for managing sedation in these patients is beyond the scope of this review and is the subject of forthcoming expert guidelines.[29] This section, therefore, focuses on 2 key components of sedation management that can improve brain function: performing coordinated daily spontaneous awakening and spontaneous breathing trials (awake and breathing coordination), and avoiding administration of benzodiazepines.

The daily cessation of sedatives (whether given by infusion or bolus doses) combined with daily spontaneous breathing trials in the Awakening and Breathing Controlled (ABC) trial resulted in a significant decrease in the number of days patients had acute brain dysfunction in comparison with the control group.[5] Specifically, duration of coma was significantly reduced, whereas duration of delirium was not. When interpreting these findings, one must consider that delirium cannot be assessed in patients who are comatose. Thus, a reduction in coma among patients in the intervention group during the first few days following initiation of the ABC protocol meant that a higher number of patients could be assessed and diagnosed with delirium; that is, delirium was no longer masked by sedative-induced coma, resulting in a biased comparison of delirium duration. Although the overall duration of delirium was similar between the two groups, patients in the intervention group were delirious earlier in their ICU stay and had resolution of acute brain dysfunction sooner than patients in the usual care group. Thus, compared with more traditional sedation strategies, daily interruption of sedatives as part of the Wake Up and Breathe protocol studied in the ABC trial reduces the overall number of days ICU patients have acute brain dysfunction (coma plus delirium) and speeds recovery of normal brain function.

Not only the general approach by which sedatives are administered and discontinued in the ICU, but also the type of sedatives administered, can affect brain dysfunction. Benzodiazepines have been associated with delirium in several studies across multiple ICU populations. Pandharipande and colleagues[30] determined that receiving lorazepam was independently associated with risk of delirium the next day in a dose-dependent manner, such that patients who received 20 mg or more on a given day were nearly all delirious the following day (with the exception of those who were comatose and could not be assessed for delirium). Similarly, after adjusting for potential confounders in a population of surgical and trauma ICU patients, receipt of midazolam was associated with a 2.75-fold increase in the odds of developing delirium.[7] Thus, one way to prevent delirium in the ICU may be to avoid administering benzodiazepines for routine sedation.

Although numerous randomized trials have demonstrated faster awakening times from sedation and shorter duration of mechanical ventilation among ICU patients sedated with alternative sedatives (eg, propofol or dexmedetomidine) rather than benzodiazepines, only 3 trials have specifically measured delirium on a daily basis when comparing a benzodiazepine with an alternative sedative.[6,31,32] The MENDS (Maximizing the Efficacy of targeted sedation and reducing Neurologic Dysfunction) trial randomized mechanically ventilated medical/surgical ICU patients to sedation with lorazepam versus dexmedetomidine for up to 5 days, and found that patients in the dexmedetomidine group had a median of 4 more days alive and free of delirium or coma compared with those sedated with lorazepam.[6] In addition, after the day of randomization, the daily prevalence of delirium was significantly lower for patients in the dexmedetomidine group than in those in the lorazepam group (**Fig. 2**). In a second randomized trial comparing dexmedetomidine with a benzodiazepine, the SEDCOM (Safety and Efficacy or Dexmedetomidine COmpared with Midazolam) trial, patients sedated with midazolam had a 23% higher delirium prevalence than those receiving

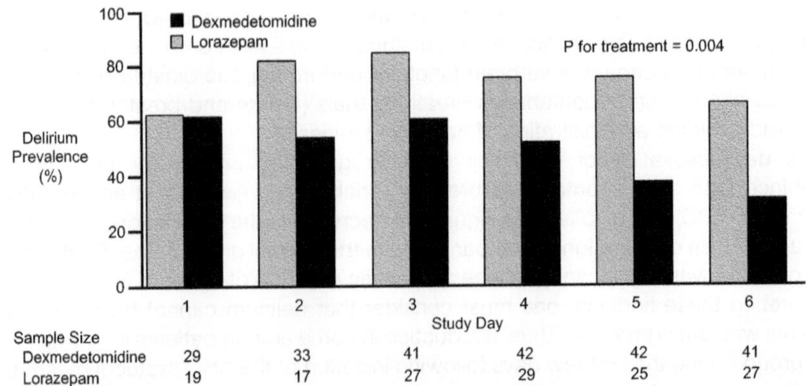

Fig. 2. In the MENDS trial, dexmedetomidine significantly reduced the prevalence of delirium over time. The sample size changed with study day as patients were extubated, died, were discharged from the ICU, or did not have delirium assessed. (*From* Pandharipande PP, Sanders RD, Girard TD, et al. Effect of dexmedetomidine versus lorazepam on outcome in patients with sepsis: an a priori-designed analysis of the MENDS randomized controlled trial. Crit Care 2010;14(2):R38; with permission.)

dexmedetomidine.[31] In another trial, Maldonado and colleagues[32] randomized patients undergoing elective cardiac valve operations to postoperative sedation with dexmedetomidine, midazolam, or propofol, and found that the incidence of delirium in the dexmedetomidine group was significantly lower than in either the midazolam or propofol groups. By contrast, the recently published MIDEX trial compared dexmedetomidine with midazolam and reported that a composite outcome of agitation, anxiety, and delirium measured at a single point in time 48 hours after the cessation of sedative infusion was not different between the midazolam and dexmedetomidine groups.[33] A simultaneously conducted trial comparing dexmedetomidine with propofol (the PRODEX trial) also found no difference between groups in agitation, anxiety, and delirium 48 hours after sedative discontinuation, but neither MIDEX nor PRODEX is informative regarding delirium given that the outcome was assessed only once during these 45-day trials. The findings of the randomized trials that implemented granular delirium measurements indicate that the avoidance of benzodiazepines is an important strategy when seeking to both prevent delirium and reduce its duration.

Preventing Delirium Through Pain Management

Pain is a modifiable risk factor for delirium, and inadequate pain control is a frequent cause for agitation in the ICU. When pain is not assessed and treated, patients may be inappropriately given a sedative medication rather than an analgesic medication. Payen and colleagues[34] found that ICU patients who were assessed for pain were less likely to receive sedatives, particularly deliriogenic benzodiazepines, and more likely to receive analgesic medications (nonopioids or opioids) than those who never had a pain assessment.

The relationship between and opioid analgesics and delirium in the ICU may appear complex when examining the literature, given the seemingly conflicting results of observational studies. However, these results yield a consistent message when understood in light of the dual effects of opioid medications: analgesia and sedation. In ICU populations where opioids are used most often used to treat pain (eg, in trauma and burn ICU populations), treatment with opioid analgesics has been associated with a reduced risk of delirium.[7,35] Conversely, in ICU populations, such as in general medical and surgical ICU populations, where opioids are frequently used for sedation (either alone or in conjunction with other sedating medications, particularly benzodiazepines), treatment with opioid analgesics has been associated with an increased risk of delirium, especially when their use induces coma.[3,7,13,36,37]

In summary, these data suggest that opioids used to treat pain are protective against the development of delirium, whereas those used at doses high enough to cause sedation may increase the risk of delirium. Therefore, patients should undergo regular pain assessments, and when pain is detected effective doses of an analgesic medication should be given, taking care to avoid inducing heavy sedation.

Preventing Delirium Through Early Mobilization of ICU Patients

Immobility has been identified as a risk factor for delirium in multiple non-ICU studies.[21,22] Until recently, however, conventional wisdom held that critically ill patients, particularly those receiving mechanical ventilation, were too sick to participate in physical rehabilitation and mobility. In recent years this belief has been challenged, and the safety and efficacy of providing ICU patients with physical rehabilitation at the earliest stages of their illness has been demonstrated.[38–44]

Two studies of early mobilization assessed patients for delirium to examine the relationship between early mobility/physical rehabilitation and delirium.[41,42] Schweickert and colleagues,[41] for example, performed a randomized trial of early physical and occupational therapy (PT/OT) beginning within the first 72 hours of endotracheal intubation and assessed patients for delirium on a daily basis. Patients in the early PT/OT group had half the number of days of delirium while in the ICU in comparison with those receiving usual care. A similar finding was noted in a quality-improvement project at Johns Hopkins Hospital, where an emphasis was placed on reducing deep sedation and increasing the number of patients managed with early mobility. In the year following the implementation of this quality-improvement project, patients spent more days without delirium and coma than those managed before initiation of the project.[42] These data suggest a role for early mobility in the reduction of the duration of delirium among critically ill patients. Further study is needed to determine whether these interventions can prevent the development of delirium.

Preventing Delirium Through Improving Sleep in the ICU

Sleep deprivation is nearly universal for ICU patients, with the average ICU patient sleeping between 2 and 8 hours in a 24-hour period.[45] Sleep in the ICU is characterized by frequent interruptions and almost half occurs during the daytime hours; thus, very little sleep in the ICU is restorative, rapid-eye-movement (REM) sleep.[45,46] Reasons for poor sleep in the ICU include the continuous cycle of alarms, lights, beepers, care-related interruptions, pain, anxiety, and ventilator dyssynchrony.[47] In addition, critically ill patients are frequently treated with medications that disrupt REM sleep including sedatives (particularly benzodiazepines), analgesics, vasopressors, β-agonists, and corticosteroids.[48] The association between sleep deprivation and delirium is unclear, as both can present with symptoms of inattention, fluctuating mental status, memory impairment, and cognitive dysfunction.[49,50] Nevertheless, nonpharmacologic and pharmacologic sleep-promoting interventions for ICU patients have been studied, but only one trial assessed whether improving sleep reduces delirium in the ICU.[51–53] Van Rompaey and colleagues[51] randomized adult ICU patients to nighttime earplug use or no earplugs. Patients sleeping with earplugs reported better sleep during the first night in the ICU, and fewer patients in this group demonstrated delirium or mild confusion during the 5-night study period. Thus, although further study is needed on potential mechanisms linking sleep deprivation and delirium, and future trials of interventions seeking to improve the quantity and quality of sleep in the ICU are necessary and should include delirium measurement as outcomes, available evidence suggests that enhancing sleep through nonpharmacologic means can reduce the incidence of delirium. Noise-reduction strategies (such as earplugs), normalizing day-night illumination, minimizing care-related interventions during normal sleeping hours, and interventions promoting patient comfort and relaxation are low risk and often inexpensive, and should be implemented to prevent delirium.

Preventing Delirium Through Pharmacologic Interventions

Pharmacologic interventions to prevent delirium are attractive, given the ease with which a medication can be administered in comparison with the implementation of nonpharmacologic interventions such as early mobility and sleep-enhancing protocols, but there are currently no medications approved by the US Food and Drug Administration for the prevention or treatment of delirium. Of those studies of pharmacologic agents to prevent delirium have been performed, most included only cardiac-surgery patients or postoperative hip-fracture patients; because these populations rarely require long-term ICU treatment, findings from these studies may not be generalizable to medical and surgical ICU populations.[27,54–56] Two studies, however, have specifically explored the role of antipsychotics for primary delirium prevention among critically ill, noncardiac-surgery patients. The MIND (Modifying the Incidence of Neurologic Dysfunction) study randomized mechanically ventilated patients admitted to medical, surgical, or trauma ICUs across 6 institutions to receive haloperidol, ziprasidone, or placebo, with treatment beginning immediately after enrollment (some patients were already delirious, whereas others were not).[57] Compared with placebo, neither of the antipsychotic drugs studied increased the number of days patients had normal brain function (ie, were alive without coma or delirium). By contrast, Wang and colleagues[58] randomized postoperative, noncardiac-surgery patients aged 65 years and older to prophylactic haloperidol or placebo, and found that patients receiving haloperidol prophylaxis were less likely to develop delirium during the 7-day study period. One major difference between these 2 studies, which may explain their disparate findings, is the severity of illness in study populations; the Wang study enrolled elective surgery patients who were not severely ill, whereas the MIND study included only critically ill patients on mechanical ventilation for acute respiratory failure. To date, these studies represent the only 2 placebo-controlled trials of antipsychotics for the prevention of ICU delirium. Although a large placebo-controlled trial of antipsychotics for the treatment delirium is ongoing,[59] more data are needed before antipsychotics can be routinely recommended for the prevention of delirium in the ICU.

Three studies of pharmacologic interventions intended to treat delirium during critical illness are worthy of mention. In an early trial, haloperidol was compared with the atypical antipsychotic olanzapine in delirious, critically ill adults and demonstrated a similar rate of improvement in delirium index scores, but no placebo comparator was used.[60] A second small trial compared quetiapine with placebo among patients already receiving haloperidol, and found faster resolution of delirium symptoms among patients treated with quetiapine.[61] The third, randomized trial compared the efficacy of adding rivastigmine, a cholinesterase inhibitor, to haloperidol for the treatment of delirious ICU patients.[62] This trial was stopped early because of higher mortality among those patients receiving rivastigmine.

Thus, prophylactic administration of antipsychotics to prevent delirium may be indicated in elderly postoperative patients, but there is no evidence currently supporting this approach in the broader population of critically ill patients. Routine treatment of delirium with antipsychotics is the subject of ongoing study. Current evidence from one small study suggests a potential benefit of the addition of quetiapine to haloperidol, but these findings need corroboration in a larger, multicenter trial. Finally, cholinesterase inhibitors should not be used to treat delirious patients in the ICU.

The ABCDE Approach to Combining Best Practices to Prevent Delirium

Delirium in the ICU is frequently multifactorial, so it is unlikely that a single intervention can prevent or reduce delirium with regularity. Therefore, a bundled approach combining evidence-based practices in sedation management, ventilator weaning, delirium management, and early mobility and exercise, which is referred to as the ABCDE approach, has been proposed to improve multiple outcomes, including preventing and reducing the duration of delirium in the ICU (**Table 2**).[63–65] The ABCDE approach combines Awakening and Breathing Coordination for liberation from sedation and mechanical ventilation, Choosing sedatives that are less likely to increase the risk of delirium, Delirium management, and finally, Early mobility and Exercise. In addition to potential positive effects on delirium, components of the ABCDEs are individually associated with numerous improvements in outcomes, including shorter duration of mechanical ventilation, shorter length of stay in the ICU and hospital, improved functional outcomes, and improved survival.

Table 2
The ABCDEs of delirium prevention

Intervention	Improved Delirium Outcomes	Other Improved Outcomes
Awakening and Breathing Coordination *Combine daily spontaneous awakening trials with daily spontaneous breathing trials*	Shorter coma duration	Shorter duration of mechanical ventilation Shorter length of stay in ICU and hospital Improved survival at 1 y
Choice of sedative agents *Avoid benzodiazepines*	Lower prevalence of delirium Shorter duration of acute brain dysfunction (duration or coma)	Shorter duration of mechanical ventilation Greater sedation accuracy (more time at target level)
Delirium Monitoring and Management *Frequently monitor patients for delirium and address modifiable/preventable risk factors and provide nonpharmacologic interventions (reorientation, cognitive stimulation, assess and treat pain, reduce sleep interruption and nonpharmacologic sleep enhancement)*	Increased detection of delirium	
Early Mobility and Exercise *Mobilize patients out of bed early in the course of their critical illness*	Shorter duration of delirium	Increased return to functional independence at hospital discharge Shorter length of stay in ICU and hospital Decreased odds of death/rehospitalization

Awakening and breathing coordination

As discussed earlier, daily spontaneous awakening trials coordinated with daily spontaneous breathing trials were associated with a significant decrease in the overall duration of acute brain dysfunction in the ABC trial. Furthermore, patients managed with this strategy were extubated an average of 3 days sooner and were discharged from the ICU and hospital an average of 4 days sooner than those managed with usual care. Remarkably, the coordination of daily spontaneous awakening trials and spontaneous breathing trials was associated with a 14% reduction in mortality at 1-year follow-up.[5]

Choice of sedative agent

The choice of sedating agent can similarly have important implications not only for delirium but also duration of mechanical ventilation and other outcomes. Both the MENDS and SEDCOM trials described earlier reported a decrease in delirium in the groups treated with dexmedetomidine compared with those treated with benzodiazepines. The SEDCOM trial also reported a 2-day reduction in time to extubation among patients treated with dexmedetomidine rather than midazolam. In the MIDEX study, treatment with dexmedetomidine also led to a shorter duration of mechanical ventilation than sedation with midazolam.[33] In addition, an a priori specified subgroup analysis of patients with severe sepsis in the MENDS trial demonstrated that septic patients treated with dexmedetomidine had an increased number of ventilator-free days and a significantly lower 28-day mortality than septic patients treated with lorazepam.[66] Thus, treatment with sedative agents other than benzodiazepines is associated with reductions in delirium development as well as reductions in the duration of mechanical ventilation.

Monitoring and management of delirium

Delirium is commonly overlooked by ICU practitioners unless a validated screening tool is used to detect its presence.[67,68] Clinicians should therefore monitor patients for the presence of delirium using a delirium screening tool designed for use in the ICU. Recent expert guidelines advocate the use of the Confusion Assessment Method for the ICU (CAM-ICU) or the Intensive Care Unit Delirium Screening Checklist (ICDSC).[29] Whereas delirium monitoring is not associated with preventing the syndrome or shortening its duration, the presence of a positive screening test alerts the clinician to look for a reversible or treatable risk factor (see **Table 1**). Only after identifying and treating reversible causes and attempting nonpharmacologic management of patients at risk for or with delirium (eg, addressing sleep deprivation, immobility, dehydration, visual and hearing impairment) should the clinician consider pharmacologic intervention.

Early mobility and exercise

As already discussed, early physical rehabilitation and early mobility have beneficial effects on reducing delirium. Early mobility is associated with numerous other beneficial outcomes in addition to effects on cognition. Morris and colleagues[39] found that patients treated with an early mobility protocol were out of bed nearly 1 week earlier, were discharged from the ICU 2 days earlier, and were discharged from the hospital 3.5 days earlier than those receiving usual care. The effects of this intervention were long lasting, as patients who were treated by the early mobility team while in the ICU were less likely to be readmitted to the hospital or die in the year following their index hospitalization.[40] Schweickert and colleagues[41] conducted the first randomized trial of early physical and occupational therapy in ICU patients, during which patients in the intervention group first received therapy within 72 hours of intubation, nearly 6 days sooner than those in the usual-care group. In addition to a reduction in duration of delirium, receipt of early PT/OT was associated with an increased probability of return to baseline functional status at the time of hospital discharge. Finally, Needham and colleagues[42] reported a 2-day shorter average length of ICU stay and a 3-day shorter length of stay in hospital compared with the previous year, following the implementation of a quality-improvement initiative that emphasized freeing patients from deep sedation, and routine consultation of physical therapy, occupational therapy, and psychiatry for the critically ill.

SUMMARY

Delirium in the ICU is exceedingly common, and risk factors for delirium among the critically ill are nearly ubiquitous. Nevertheless, addressing modifiable risk factors including sedation management, deliriogenic medications, immobility, and sleep disruption can help to prevent and reduce the duration of this deadly syndrome. The ABCDE approach to critical care is a bundled approach that can be implemented by clinicians for many patients treated in their ICUs to prevent the adverse outcomes associated with delirium and critical illness.

REFERENCES

1. American Psychiatric Association. Diagnostic and statistical manual of mental disorders. Fourth edition, text revision. Washington, DC: American Psychiatric Association; 2000.
2. Ely EW, Inouye SK, Bernard GR, et al. Delirium in mechanically ventilated patients: validity and reliability of the confusion assessment method for the intensive care unit (CAM-ICU). JAMA 2001;286(21):2703–10.
3. Dubois MJ, Bergeron N, Dumont M, et al. Delirium in an intensive care unit: a study of risk factors. Intensive Care Med 2001;27(8):1297–304.
4. Bergeron N, Dubois MJ, Dumont M, et al. Intensive Care Delirium Screening Checklist: evaluation of a new screening tool. Intensive Care Med 2001;27(5):859–64.
5. Girard TD, Kress JP, Fuchs BD, et al. Efficacy and safety of a paired sedation and ventilator weaning protocol for mechanically ventilated patients in intensive care (Awakening and Breathing Controlled trial): a randomised controlled trial. Lancet 2008;371(9607):126–34.
6. Pandharipande PP, Pun BT, Herr DL, et al. Effect of sedation with dexmedetomidine vs lorazepam on acute brain dysfunction in mechanically ventilated patients: the MENDS randomized controlled trial. JAMA 2007;298(22):2644–53.
7. Pandharipande P, Cotton BA, Shintani A, et al. Prevalence and risk factors for development of delirium in surgical and trauma intensive care unit patients. J Trauma 2008;65(1):34–41.
8. Guenther U, Popp J, Koecher L, et al. Validity and reliability of the CAM-ICU flowsheet to diagnose delirium in surgical ICU patients. J Crit Care 2010;25(1):144–51.
9. Micek ST, Anand NJ, Laible BR, et al. Delirium as detected by the CAM-ICU predicts restraint use among mechanically ventilated medical patients. Crit Care Med 2005;33(6):1260–5.
10. Shehabi Y, Riker RR, Bokesch PM, et al. Delirium duration and mortality in lightly sedated, mechanically ventilated intensive care unit patients. Crit Care Med 2010;38(12):2311–8.
11. Ely EW, Gautam S, Margolin R, et al. The impact of delirium in the intensive care unit on hospital length of stay. Intensive Care Med 2001;27(12):1892–900.
12. Ely EW, Shintani A, Truman B, et al. Delirium as a predictor of mortality in mechanically ventilated patients in the intensive care unit. JAMA 2004;291(14):1753–62.
13. Ouimet S, Kavanagh BP, Gottfried SB, et al. Incidence, risk factors and consequences of ICU delirium. Intensive Care Med 2007;33(1):66–73.
14. Thomason JW, Shintani A, Peterson JF, et al. Intensive care unit delirium is an independent predictor of longer hospital stay: a prospective analysis of 261 non-ventilated patients. Crit Care 2005;9(4):R375–81.
15. Milbrandt EB, Deppen S, Harrison PL, et al. Costs associated with delirium in mechanically ventilated patients. Crit Care Med 2004;32(4):955–62.
16. Lin SM, Liu CY, Wang CH, et al. The impact of delirium on the survival of mechanically ventilated patients. Crit Care Med 2004;32(11):2254–9.
17. Pisani MA, Kong SY, Kasl SV, et al. Days of delirium are associated with 1-year mortality in an older intensive care unit population. Am J Respir Crit Care Med 2009;180(11):1092–7.
18. Van Rompaey B, Schuurmans MJ, Shortridge-Baggett LM, et al. Long term outcome after delirium in the intensive care unit. J Clin Nurs 2009;18(23):3349–57.
19. Girard TD, Jackson JC, Pandharipande PP, et al. Delirium as a predictor of long-term cognitive impairment in survivors of critical illness. Crit Care Med 2010;38(7):1513–20.

20. Brummel NE, Jackson JC, Torres R, et al. Does duration of ICU delirium predict long-term functional impairment? Am J Respir Crit Care Med 2011;183:A2653.
21. Inouye SK, Charpentier PA. Precipitating factors for delirium in hospitalized elderly persons. Predictive model and interrelationship with baseline vulnerability. JAMA 1996;275(11):852–7.
22. Inouye SK, Bogardus ST Jr, Charpentier PA, et al. A multicomponent intervention to prevent delirium in hospitalized older patients. N Engl J Med 1999;340(9): 669–76.
23. Martinez FT, Tobar C, Beddings CI, et al. Preventing delirium in an acute hospital using a non-pharmacological intervention. Age Ageing 2012;41(5):629–34.
24. Marcantonio ER, Flacker JM, Wright RJ, et al. Reducing delirium after hip fracture: a randomized trial. J Am Geriatr Soc 2001;49(5):516–22.
25. Kalisvaart KJ, de Jonghe JF, Bogaards MJ, et al. Haloperidol prophylaxis for elderly hip-surgery patients at risk for delirium: a randomized placebo-controlled study. J Am Geriatr Soc 2005;53(10):1658–66.
26. Larsen KA, Kelly SE, Stern TA, et al. Administration of olanzapine to prevent postoperative delirium in elderly joint-replacement patients: a randomized, controlled trial. Psychosomatics 2010;51(5):409–18.
27. Prakanrattana U, Prapaitrakool S. Efficacy of risperidone for prevention of postoperative delirium in cardiac surgery. Anaesth Intensive Care 2007;35(5):714–9.
28. Patel RP, Gambrell M, Speroff T, et al. Delirium and sedation in the intensive care unit: survey of behaviors and attitudes of 1384 healthcare professionals. Crit Care Med 2009;37(3):825–32.
29. Barr J, Fraser GL, Puntillo K, et al. Clinical practice guidelines for the management of pain, agitation, and delirium in adult patients in the intensive care unit. Critical Care Medicine, in press.
30. Pandharipande P, Shintani A, Peterson J, et al. Lorazepam is an independent risk factor for transitioning to delirium in intensive care unit patients. Anesthesiology 2006;104(1):21–6.
31. Riker RR, Shehabi Y, Bokesch PM, et al. Dexmedetomidine vs midazolam for sedation of critically ill patients: a randomized trial. JAMA 2009;301(5):489–99.
32. Maldonado JR, Wysong A, van der Starre PJ, et al. Dexmedetomidine and the reduction of postoperative delirium after cardiac surgery. Psychosomatics 2009;50(3):206–17.
33. Jakob SM, Ruokonen E, Grounds RM, et al. Dexmedetomidine vs midazolam or propofol for sedation during prolonged mechanical ventilation: two randomized controlled trials. JAMA 2012;307(11):1151–60.
34. Payen JF, Bosson JL, Chanques G, et al. Pain assessment is associated with decreased duration of mechanical ventilation in the intensive care unit: a post Hoc analysis of the DOLOREA study. Anesthesiology 2009;111(6):1308–16.
35. Agarwal V, O'Neill PJ, Cotton BA, et al. Prevalence and risk factors for development of delirium in burn intensive care unit patients. J Burn Care Res 2010;31(5):706–15.
36. Van Rompaey B, Elseviers MM, Schuurmans MJ, et al. Risk factors for delirium in intensive care patients: a prospective cohort study. Crit Care 2009;13(3):R77.
37. Pisani MA, Murphy TE, Araujo KL, et al. Benzodiazepine and opioid use and the duration of intensive care unit delirium in an older population. Crit Care Med 2009; 37(1):177–83.
38. Bailey P, Thomsen GE, Spuhler VJ, et al. Early activity is feasible and safe in respiratory failure patients. Crit Care Med 2007;35(1):139–45.
39. Morris PE, Goad A, Thompson C, et al. Early intensive care unit mobility therapy in the treatment of acute respiratory failure. Crit Care Med 2008;36(8):2238–43.

40. Morris PE, Griffin L, Berry M, et al. Receiving early mobility during an intensive care unit admission is a predictor of improved outcomes in acute respiratory failure. Am J Med Sci 2011;341(5):373–7.
41. Schweickert WD, Pohlman MC, Pohlman AS, et al. Early physical and occupational therapy in mechanically ventilated, critically ill patients: a randomised controlled trial. Lancet 2009;373(9678):1874–82.
42. Needham DM, Korupolu R, Zanni JM, et al. Early physical medicine and rehabilitation for patients with acute respiratory failure: a quality improvement project. Arch Phys Med Rehabil 2010;91(4):536–42.
43. Needham DM, Korupolu R. Rehabilitation quality improvement in an intensive care unit setting: implementation of a quality improvement model. Top Stroke Rehabil 2010;17(4):271–81.
44. Needham DM. Mobilizing patients in the intensive care unit: improving neuromuscular weakness and physical function. JAMA 2008;300(14):1685–90.
45. Cooper AB, Thornley KS, Young GB, et al. Sleep in critically ill patients requiring mechanical ventilation. Chest 2000;117(3):809–18.
46. Gabor JY, Cooper AB, Crombach SA, et al. Contribution of the intensive care unit environment to sleep disruption in mechanically ventilated patients and healthy subjects. Am J Respir Crit Care Med 2003;167(5):708–15.
47. Hardin KA. Sleep in the ICU: potential mechanisms and clinical implications. Chest 2009;136(1):284–94.
48. Bourne RS, Mills GH. Sleep disruption in critically ill patients—pharmacological considerations. Anaesthesia 2004;59(4):374–84.
49. Mistraletti G, Carloni E, Cigada M, et al. Sleep and delirium in the intensive care unit. Minerva Anestesiol 2008;74(6):329–33.
50. Weinhouse GL, Schwab RJ, Watson PL, et al. Bench-to-bedside review: delirium in ICU patients—importance of sleep deprivation. Crit Care 2009;13(6): 234.
51. Van Rompaey B, Elseviers MM, Van Drom W, et al. The effect of earplugs during the night on the onset of delirium and sleep perception: a randomized controlled trial in intensive care patients. Crit Care 2012;16(3):R73.
52. Hu RF, Jiang XY, Zeng YM, et al. Effects of earplugs and eye masks on nocturnal sleep, melatonin and cortisol in a simulated intensive care unit environment. Crit Care 2010;14(2):R66.
53. Bourne RS, Mills GH, Minelli C. Melatonin therapy to improve nocturnal sleep in critically ill patients: encouraging results from a small randomised controlled trial. Crit Care 2008;12(2):R52.
54. Gamberini M, Bolliger D, Lurati Buse GA, et al. Rivastigmine for the prevention of postoperative delirium in elderly patients undergoing elective cardiac surgery—a randomized controlled trial. Crit Care Med 2009;37(5):1762–8.
55. Hudetz JA, Patterson KM, Iqbal Z, et al. Ketamine attenuates delirium after cardiac surgery with cardiopulmonary bypass. J Cardiothorac Vasc Anesth 2009;23(5): 651–7.
56. Shehabi Y, Grant P, Wolfenden H, et al. Prevalence of delirium with dexmedetomidine compared with morphine based therapy after cardiac surgery: a randomized controlled trial (DEXmedetomidine COmpared to Morphine—DEXCOM Study). Anesthesiology 2009;111(5):1075–84.
57. Girard TD, Pandharipande PP, Carson SS, et al. Feasibility, efficacy, and safety of antipsychotics for intensive care unit delirium: the MIND randomized, placebo-controlled trial. Crit Care Med 2010;38(2):428–37.

58. Wang W, Li HL, Wang DX, et al. Haloperidol prophylaxis decreases delirium incidence in elderly patients after noncardiac surgery: a randomized controlled trial*. Crit Care Med 2012;40(3):731–9.
59. Ely EW. MIND-ICU Study: delirium and dementia in veterans surviving ICU care. http://clinicaltrials.gov/ct2/show/NCT01211522. Accessed August 31, 2012.
60. Skrobik YK, Bergeron N, Dumont M, et al. Olanzapine vs haloperidol: treating delirium in a critical care setting. Intensive Care Med 2004;30(3):444–9.
61. Devlin JW, Roberts RJ, Fong JJ, et al. Efficacy and safety of quetiapine in critically ill patients with delirium: a prospective, multicenter, randomized, double-blind, placebo-controlled pilot study. Crit Care Med 2010;38(2):419–27.
62. van Eijk MM, Roes KC, Honing ML, et al. Effect of rivastigmine as an adjunct to usual care with haloperidol on duration of delirium and mortality in critically ill patients: a multicentre, double-blind, placebo-controlled randomised trial. Lancet 2010;376(9755):1829–37.
63. Morandi A, Brummel NE, Ely EW. Sedation, delirium and mechanical ventilation: the 'ABCDE' approach. Curr Opin Crit Care 2011;17(1):43–9.
64. Vasilevskis EE, Ely EW, Speroff T, et al. Reducing iatrogenic risks: ICU-acquired delirium and weakness—crossing the quality chasm. Chest 2010;138(5):1224–33.
65. Vasilevskis EE, Pandharipande PP, Girard TD, et al. A screening, prevention, and restoration model for saving the injured brain in intensive care unit survivors. Crit Care Med 2010;38(Suppl 10):S683–91.
66. Pandharipande PP, Sanders RD, Girard TD, et al. Effect of dexmedetomidine versus lorazepam on outcome in patients with sepsis: an a priori-designed analysis of the MENDS randomized controlled trial. Crit Care 2010;14(2):R38.
67. Spronk PE, Riekerk B, Hofhuis J, et al. Occurrence of delirium is severely underestimated in the ICU during daily care. Intensive Care Med 2009;35(7):1276–80.
68. van Eijk MM, van Marum RJ, Klijn IA, et al. Comparison of delirium assessment tools in a mixed intensive care unit. Crit Care Med 2009;37(6):1881–5.

Sedation and Mobility

Changing the Paradigm

John P. Kress, MD

KEYWORDS

- Respiratory failure • Physical therapy • Occupational therapy • Mobilization
- Mechanical ventilation • ICU-acquired weakness • Critical illness myopathy
- Sedation

KEY POINTS

- Intensive care unit (ICU) acquired weakness is a common complication in survivors with respiratory failure.
- Deconditioning occurs rapidly in patients who require mechanical ventilation.
- Recent evidence has led to a shift away from deep sedation in mechanically ventilated patients.
- Early mobility is possible in patients who are alert, even during mechanical ventilation.
- Early mobility has been associated with significant improvements in ICU patient outcomes.

Critically ill patients frequently present in extremes of physiologic derangement, and intensive care unit (ICU) clinicians often prioritize their attention to recovery and maintenance of homeostasis compatible with survival. As such, acute organ system failure (eg, cardiovascular, pulmonary, renal) traditionally has received the highest priority, particularly during early phases of critical illness. Patients with respiratory failure requiring mechanical ventilation are certainly the most challenging in this regard.[1] Most trials in critically ill patients have focused on short-term end points, which do not address patients' longer-term morbidities or impairments in quality of life and functional status. Yet survival from critical illness has improved greatly over the past 20 years. As an example, mortality from acute respiratory distress syndrome (ARDS) has been reported to be in the 20% range in several recent trials. This finding is a substantial improvement from the greater than 50% mortality reported in trials just 20 years ago.[2] With this improved survival has come a new burden of profound and persistent impairments in physical (eg, muscle weakness) and cognitive (eg, memory) function.[3–5] The rehabilitation process for these patients is often long and incomplete.

Support: None.
Section of Pulmonary and Critical Care, Department of Medicine, University of Chicago, 5841 South Maryland, MC 6026, Chicago, IL 60637, USA
E-mail address: jkress@medicine.bsd.uchicago.edu

Crit Care Clin 29 (2013) 67–75
http://dx.doi.org/10.1016/j.ccc.2012.10.001 **criticalcare.theclinics.com**
0749-0704/13/$ – see front matter

Research addressing the issues surrounding recovery after critical illness has only recently begun to appear in the literature.

Reports of recovery from critical illness and respiratory failure note severe physical deconditioning accompanied by weight loss, profound weakness, and functional impairment.[6–9] A growing literature identifies neuropathies and myopathies in patients, which can be described categorically as ICU-acquired weakness.[10] Although ICU-acquired weakness may be either *neuropathic* or *myopathic*, it is clear that there is considerable overlap between these entities.[11–14] *Critical illness polyneuropathy*, first described more than 20 years ago,[15] is characterized by a primary axonal degeneration, typically beginning in distal axons and affecting motor nerves more than sensory nerves.[16] Demyelination is not seen in this condition. Electrophysiological studies show reduction in amplitudes of compound motor and sensory nerve action potentials, with preservation of conduction velocity. A *critical illness myopathy* presents with generalized muscle weakness but preserved sensory function. Although the mechanisms are poorly understood,[17] preliminary evidence suggests that muscle injury from systemic inflammation[18,19] along with deconditioning from immobility[12,20] may be important. Catabolism with skeletal muscle proteolysis and atrophy are frequently observed in ICU patients and also may contribute to ICU-acquired weakness. The clinical syndrome of ICU-acquired weakness is complex and multifactorial, and the resulting debilitation is devastating for a large fraction of ICU survivors.[21] This debilitation is particularly common in those suffering from ARDS, sepsis, and/or the systemic inflammatory response syndrome.[22,23]

For many decades, the standard approach to caring for critically ill patients has been to subject such patients to complete bed rest.[24] This practice is particularly so in those with respiratory failure requiring mechanical ventilation. These patients are typically subjected to liberal administration of sedative and analgesic drugs, a care strategy that leads to a state of physical and mental immobilization. It is interesting that care of hospitalized patients is focused on bed rest (indeed, the size of a hospital is measured with a currency of beds); yet, the harmful effects of complete bed rest in the hospital have been recognized and described as early as the 1940s.[25,26] Intensive care physicians are accustomed to providing advanced technologies to support failing organs. There are ventilators for respiratory failure, dialytic therapies for kidney failure, ventricular assist devices for heart failure, and, of course, transplantation for many different organ failures. Yet the brain and neuromuscular systems have no available support systems. On reflection, it might seem to an outsider that the brain and neuromuscular systems have been treated as second-class citizens in the ICU while we struggle to keep the more vital organ systems functional. Connecting patients to artificial life support systems may require that they be forced to accept these therapies, which by their nature may be noxious and invasive. The solution of deep sedation is not without cost, however. More recently, clinicians have begun to rethink the perception that deep sedation to fully take over for failing bodily functions is wise or necessary.[27,28] The notion that hospitalization, even in the ICU, mandates full bed rest is changing.[29]

In recent literature, there has been a growing focus on long-term outcomes in ICU survivors, particularly those with respiratory failure. Margaret Herridge and colleagues[7] reported one of the early reports of outcomes in ARDS survivors nearly 10 years ago. This group of investigators evaluated ARDS survivors for physical as well as mental functional problems 1 year after ICU discharge. The group of 109 survivors was young (median age 45 years), yet every patient reported loss of muscle bulk, proximal muscle weakness, and fatigue. A year after their ICU discharge, half of the cohort was unemployed. A follow-up report of the same group of ARDS survivors 5 years from hospital discharge noted ongoing physical limitations. The cohort of surviving patients (now reduced to 64 in total) had subnormal scores on 6-minute walk tests and physical component scores on the 36-Item Short Form Health Survey (SF-36).[30] Their mental component scores had returned to a low-normal level by the end of this 5-year period.

The effect of prolonged physical immobility on subsequent neuromuscular function has received a relative paucity of scientific investigation. Animal models of prolonged immobility report a loss of molecular motor protein myosin and subsequent impairment of muscle function.[31,32] Human studies of the effects of prolonged physical immobilization, a state that is ubiquitous in the ICU, are likewise relatively rare. In 1995, Griffiths and colleagues[20] evaluated the effects of neuromuscular blockade in humans undergoing mechanical ventilation. They compared the effects of continuous passive motion of one leg with the patients' contralateral leg serving as a control; muscle fiber atrophy was prevented, and muscle DNA to protein ratios and muscle protein content were reduced less profoundly in the leg subjected to continuous passive range of motion. The investigators concluded that in critically ill patients requiring mechanical ventilation, an intervention as simple as passive muscle stretching and movement could preserve the structural architecture of the muscle fibers.

Over the last 5 years, several reports of a new approach to ICU care have been published. Armed with knowledge of the problems associated with recovery after critical illness, a paradigm shift has begun whereby the traditional approach to patient care with deep sedation and suspended animation of both mind and body have been substituted with a focus on early physical activity. This change in approach to patient care is predicated on the notion that prolonged bed rest is harmful. Physical therapists are the centerpiece of the intervention; but other clinicians, such as occupational therapists, nurses, respiratory therapists, and patient care technicians, are also involved. The notion that a patient is too sick to get out of bed is being replaced by the notion that the patient may be too sick to afford staying in bed. Accordingly, even patients who are intubated and mechanically ventilated have been undergoing mobilization therapy.

As alluded to earlier, early mobilization requires that patients are awake and able to interact with their environment. This early mobilization is clearly not feasible when patients are deeply sedated. Over the last decade, numerous studies have reported on the benefits of lighter sedation of patients undergoing mechanical ventilation.[27,28,33–35] As such, it is now feasible to expect that patients who are mechanically ventilated can actually be interactive with their environment. One of the earliest studies reporting a possible link between deep sedation and the adverse effects of the resulting immobility came from De Jonghe and colleagues.[35] His group described a before-after study whereby usual care sedation was compared with a sedation algorithm designed to improve patient alertness. The group had described an algorithm designed around the Adaptation to the Intensive Care Environment (ATICE) sedation instrument. This instrument targeted several domains: consciousness (with awakeness and consciousness subdomains) and tolerance (with calmness, ventilatory synchrony, and face relaxation subdomains). This ATICE instrument was used to direct a nursing sedation algorithm. Transitioning from usual care to an algorithm driven by the ATICE instrument led to reduced ventilator time and ICU length of stay. Most interesting from the standpoint of immobilization was the 50% reduction in pressure sores noted. This finding is very likely caused by the reduced state of immobility noted with more alert patients.

The first report of intentional physical therapy in mechanically ventilated patients was published by the group from LDS Hospital in Salt Lake City, Utah. This group, led by Bailey and colleagues,[36] reported a novel approach to the management of mechanically ventilated patients. In their special respiratory ICU, patients were routinely moved out of bed to a chair and even walked, all while still intubated. The paradigm shift involved a culture of minimal sedation and early mobilization, which was directed by a physical therapist, a respiratory therapist, a nurse, and a critical care technician. The traditional view that mechanically ventilated patients are too unstable to mobilize was challenged. Instead, mobilization started as soon as patients were responsive to verbal stimulation and had respiratory and cardiovascular stability, which was defined as ventilator settings of fraction of inspired oxygen of 0.6 or less and positive end-expiratory pressure of 10 cm H_2O or less and the absence of orthostatic hypotension and catecholamine infusions. Every protocol for mobilization, including this first one, has used a progressive approach whereby patients began with simple activities (eg, sitting at the edge of the bed) and progressed to more advanced activities, such as standing, marching in place, and walking. This progression occurred at a pace commensurate with the individual patient's tolerance. Indeed, a similar approach to mobilization is used routinely by physical therapists caring for patients in less acute settings. In this first report of mobilization in mechanically ventilated patients by Bailey and colleagues, more than 100 patients underwent 1500 activity events. Their level of activity was quite remarkable, with more than 40% of the activities occurring in those who were still intubated and mechanically ventilated. Despite this aggressive, unconventional approach, adverse events were extremely rare. This publication was the first to systematically describe the safety and feasibility of mobilization in mechanically ventilated ICU patients.

Following this descriptive study, the group from Wake Forest University, led by Peter Morris,[37] reported the first prospective comparative study of early mobilization versus usual care in ICU patients. A similar approach to minimizing sedation as described by Bailey and colleagues was used. This group used a physical therapist, a critical care nurse, and a nursing assistant. This study was prospective but not randomized. Instead, patients were assigned using a nonrandomized block allocation manner. A total of 330 patients were studied. Eighty percent of patients in the mobilization group assigned had at least one physical therapy session compared with only 47% in the usual care group. The mobilization group was out of bed 5 days sooner than the control group and had a lesser hospital stay by 2 days; both of these findings were statistically significant. Adverse events did not occur during any activity sessions. The benefits of early activity persisted in this group of patients. In a separate publication, the investigators reported that the control patients who did not receive early mobilization had a significantly higher likelihood of death or readmission to the hospital at 1 year (odds ratio, 1.77 [95% confidence interval, 1.04–3.01]).[38]

A Belgian group, led by Burtin[39] and senior author Rik Gosselink, performed a randomized controlled trial of early exercise in ICU patients, mostly from a surgical ICU. In this study, the investigators actually attached a bicycle ergometer to the foot of the bed of the patients.[39] Even though the bicycling intervention was delayed 2 weeks, the benefits were still substantial. Patients who were not aware enough to pedal the bicycle had their feet strapped to the pedals and the bicycle would pedal automatically, thus moving the patients' legs with passive range of motion. Once patients were aware, they would actively cycle the ergometer. Most patients (84%) were intubated and mechanically ventilated for at least some of their ICU stay. Strength and functional assessments were substantially better in the intervention group at the time of hospital discharge. The 6-minute walk distance was greater (196 vs 143 m, $P<.05$), the SF-36 physical function score was better (21 vs 15, $P<.05$), and the quadriceps force was better in the intervention group (2.37 vs 2.03 $N \cdot kg^{-1}$, $P<.05$). The cycling sessions were well tolerated, with only rare adverse events reported (eg, SpO_2 decrease, adverse changes in blood pressure).

A French group led by Bourdin and colleagues[40] described their experience of early mobilization in a small cohort of 20 patients. This 2009 report described a cohort that began mobilization after a median of 5 ICU days; one-third of the interventions occurred during mechanical ventilation. The group of investigators was significantly less aggressive than the previously mentioned groups in that they did not include those with shock or active renal replacement therapy and they did not include those who were receiving sedation. Mobilization included sitting up in bed, followed by moving to a chair and ultimately walking. Adverse events were again quite rare, occurring only 3% of the time.

In 2009, William Schweickert and colleagues[41] reported findings from a prospective randomized blinded trial of very early physical and occupational therapy. This study was unique in several ways. It was the first randomized trial, and blinded observers evaluated the end points. The trial also began mobilization immediately after endotracheal intubation. The investigators used data from previous work, in both animal models and humans, which suggested that neuromuscular dysfunction, at least in the diaphragm, begins very early after the inception of respiratory failure requiring mechanical ventilation.[42–44] Accordingly, the investigators began the mobilization protocol immediately, rather than waiting for several days. The intent of this trial was to initiate mobilization preemptively, before deconditioning had occurred, or at least to attempt to reduce the pace and magnitude of neuromuscular deconditioning. The study enrolled patients from medical ICUs at 2 different tertiary care academic medical centers. Patients were required to have undergone mechanical ventilation for a relatively short period of time (less than 72 hours) and to be functionally independent at baseline before their ICU admission. The randomized scheme used an intervention group that underwent a progressive physical and occupational therapy regimen focused on mobilization and achievement of occupational tasks (ie, activities of daily living [ADL]). This strategy was compared with a control group who received usual care, which did not include physical therapy until after they were extubated and preparing for discharge from the ICU. To ensure that the intervention of early mobilization was the only factor that determined whatever differences might be noted, all patients received evidence-based ICU care. These evidence-based strategies included daily sedative interruption,[33] daily spontaneous breathing trials,[45] early enteral nutrition, and tight glucose control.[46]

Each morning, all patients had their sedatives discontinued. In the intervention group, after patients were awake and able to follow instructions, a team consisting of a physical therapist and an occupational therapist began mobilizing the patients in a stepwise progressive fashion. The progressive fashion to the mobilization regimen was similar to that done with previous studies whereby patients began by sitting at the edge of the bed and progressed to dangling the legs, standing, transferring to a chair, and ultimately walking. Occupational therapists assisted these patients with ADLs, skills that are quickly lost in those who suffer respiratory failure requiring mechanical ventilation. Patients capable of performing the simpler tasks (eg, sitting at the edge of the bed) were advanced quickly to more advanced tasks on subsequent days as based on their stability and tolerance of the activities. As noted earlier, patients in the usual care control group had therapy initiated once extubated.[47–49] The primary end point of the trial was the return to functional independence at hospital discharge. Functional independence was defined a priori as the ability to perform ADLs (bathing, dressing, eating, grooming, transfer from bed to chair, toileting) and the ability to walk independently. This primary end point was chosen because it was particularly focused on a relevant outcome from the perspective of the patients. Functional independence is a necessary end point for successful discharge to home after hospitalization. Critical illness with respiratory failure requiring mechanical ventilation frequently leads to states of physical and mental deconditioning, which require extensive rehabilitation. This study reasoned that maintaining functional independence would substantially reduce this problem.

Unlike the previous studies described earlier, patients began mobilization therapy immediately after extubation, rather than the average of 5 or more days from the other trials. This practice led to the accomplishment of substantial tasks, even while still intubated. These tasks in intubated patients included bed mobility in 76%, standing in 33%, sitting in a chair in 33%, and ambulation in 15%.[50]

This immediate mobilization strategy improved functional independence at hospital discharge substantially, with 59% of the intervention group achieving this goal compared with 35% percent of the control group. The early mobilization group had more patients who were able to go directly home after hospitalization rather than a center for rehabilitation or dying (43% vs 24%, $P = .06$). The duration of mechanical ventilation was reduced (3.4 vs 6.1 days, $P = .02$), and ventilator-free days were increased (23.5 vs 21.1, $P = .05$). The early mobilization patients had better maximal walking distances (33.4 vs 0 m, $P = .004$) and greater numbers of ADLs performed at hospital discharge (6 vs 4, $P = .06$).[41] All patients underwent a daily sedative interruption protocol, and the amount of sedative drugs administered did not differ between the two groups. Despite the similar levels of sedation, ICU delirium days were reduced by 50% (2.0 vs 4.0 days, $P = .03$) in the intervention group. This finding suggests an important link between physical mobility and mental animation in critically ill patients. As noted in all of the previous published work on early mobilization, adverse events were very rare, and premature discontinuation of a therapy session occurred in only 4% of the sessions. Once again, this intervention involved a paradigm shift in which every patient was evaluated for very early mobility. The notion that a patient was not stable enough to be mobilized was replaced by an approach which considered patients with high illness acuity. For example, patients with acute lung injury made up 58% of all sessions in the study. Patients with other conditions, such as shock on vasoactive drugs, kidney failure requiring renal replacement therapy, and morbid obesity, were also subjected to early mobilization.[50]

The group from Johns Hopkins, led by Dale Needham and colleagues,[51] reported a quality-improvement project centered around early mobilization in their medical ICU patients. They used a team of physical and occupational therapists to bring a change in culture into their ICU. Patients were no longer deeply sedated; rather, they were awakened and allowed to get out of bed and start physical activity. This paradigm shift led to a dramatic reduction in sedative and opiate use and a concomitant reduction in ICU delirium. Indeed, these investigators recognized the critical importance of eliminating deep sedation to permit mobilization. After the quality-improvement project, patients received more rehabilitation treatments and accomplished a higher level of functional mobility. In conjunction with these changes, ICU length of stay decreased by an average of 2.1 days and hospital length of stay decreased by 3.1 days. The same investigators reported an observational study of patients in the medical ICU who received interactive video games, such as boxing, bowling, and balance board, as part of physical therapy. These sessions were even able to occur in patients who were undergoing mechanical ventilation.[52]

SUMMARY

A large fraction of ICU patients with respiratory failure who survive their critical illness leave the hospital with substantial neuromuscular weakness. The road to rehabilitation for these patients is long and difficult, and many never reach the level of function they enjoyed before their admission to the ICU. In light of this reality, a shift in the approach to critical care management has begun. This viewpoint has broadened the perspective of ICU care providers beyond the narrow goal of leaving the ICU alive to a broader notion focused on minimizing the complications that accompany the inherent noxious nature of ICU care. Physical and occupational therapy, although not traditionally viewed as a standard part of the care plan in mechanically ventilated patients, have demonstrated remarkable benefits in several recently published articles. It is obvious from this recent literature that mobilization of mechanically ventilated patients is feasible, safe, and carries the potential for tremendous benefit for our patients. In the future, it seems logical to evaluate which types of patients benefit most from such an aggressive mobilization approach. Furthermore, in order for widespread use of such a care model, continued focus on minimization of sedation must occur. More research is needed to identify whether there are specific groups of patients that stand to benefit from early mobilization more than others. Continued emphasis on the problems associated with deep sedation and prolonged immobility is needed to change ICU culture to one of more mental and physical animation in this group of high-risk patients.

REFERENCES

1. Rubenfeld GD, Caldwell E, Peabody E, et al. Incidence and outcomes of acute lung injury. N Engl J Med 2005;353(16):1685–93.
2. Zambon M, Vincent JL. Mortality rates for patients with acute lung injury/ARDS have decreased over time. Chest 2008;133(5):1120–7.
3. Herridge MS. Long-term outcomes after critical illness. Curr Opin Crit Care 2002;8(4):331–6.
4. Hopkins RO, Weaver LK, Collingridge D, et al. Two-year cognitive, emotional, and quality-of-life outcomes in acute respiratory distress syndrome. Am J Respir Crit Care Med 2005;171(4):340–7.
5. Rothenhausler HB, Ehrentraut S, Stoll C, et al. The relationship between cognitive performance and employment and health status in long-term survivors of the acute respiratory distress syndrome: results of an exploratory study. Gen Hosp Psychiatry 2001;23(2):90–6.
6. Angus DC, Kelley MA, Schmitz RJ, et al. Caring for the critically ill patient. Current and projected workforce requirements for care of the critically ill and patients with pulmonary disease: can we meet the requirements of an aging population? JAMA 2000;284(21):2762–70.
7. Herridge MS, Cheung AM, Tansey CM, et al. One-year outcomes in survivors of the acute respiratory distress syndrome. N Engl J Med 2003;348(8):683–93.
8. Cheung AM, Tansey CM, Tomlinson G, et al. Two-year outcomes, health care use, and costs of survivors of acute respiratory distress syndrome. Am J Respir Crit Care Med 2006;174(5):538–44.
9. Stevens RD, Dowdy DW, Michaels RK, et al. Neuromuscular dysfunction acquired in critical illness: a systematic review. Intensive Care Med 2007;33(11):1876–91.
10. De Jonghe B, Cook D, Sharshar T, et al. Acquired neuromuscular disorders in critically ill patients: a systematic review. Groupe de Reflexion et d'Etude sur les Neuromyopathies En Reanimation. Intensive Care Med 1998;24(12):1242–50.
11. Angus DC, Barnato AE, Linde-Zwirble WT, et al. Use of intensive care at the end of life in the United States: an epidemiologic study. Crit Care Med 2004;32(3):638–43.

12. Bednarik J, Lukas Z, Vondracek P. Critical illness polyneuromyopathy: the electrophysiological components of a complex entity. Intensive Care Med 2003;29(9): 1505–14.
13. Bolton CF, Breuer AC. Critical illness polyneuropathy. Muscle Nerve 1999;22(3): 419–24.
14. Bolton CF. Sepsis and the systemic inflammatory response syndrome: neuromuscular manifestations. Crit Care Med 1996;24(8):1408–16.
15. Bolton CF, Gilbert JJ, Hahn AF, et al. Polyneuropathy in critically ill patients. J Neurol Neurosurg Psychiatr 1984;47(11):1223–31.
16. Bolton CF. Neuromuscular manifestations of critical illness. Muscle Nerve 2005; 32(2):140–63.
17. Bogdanski R, Blobner M, Werner C. Critical illness polyneuropathy and myopathy: do they persist for lifetime? Crit Care Med 2003;31(4):1279–80.
18. Witt NJ, Zochodne DW, Bolton CF, et al. Peripheral nerve function in sepsis and multiple organ failure. Chest 1991;99(1):176–84.
19. Leijten FS, De Weerd AW, Poortvliet DC, et al. Critical illness polyneuropathy in multiple organ dysfunction syndrome and weaning from the ventilator. Intensive Care Med 1996;22(9):856–61.
20. Griffiths RD, Palmer TE, Helliwell T, et al. Effect of passive stretching on the wasting of muscle in the critically ill. Nutrition 1995;11(5):428–32.
21. Misak CJ. The critical care experience: a patient's view. Am J Respir Crit Care Med 2004;170(4):357–9.
22. de Letter MA, Schmitz PI, Visser LH, et al. Risk factors for the development of polyneuropathy and myopathy in critically ill patients. Crit Care Med 2001; 29(12):2281–6.
23. Latronico N. Neuromuscular alterations in the critically ill patient: critical illness myopathy, critical illness neuropathy, or both? Intensive Care Med 2003;29(9): 1411–3.
24. Petty TL. Suspended life or extending death? Chest 1998;114(2):360–1.
25. Dock W. The evil sequelae of complete bed rest. JAMA 1944;125(16):1083–5.
26. Asher RA. The dangers of going to bed. Br Med J 1947;2(4536):967.
27. Strom T, Martinussen T, Toft P. A protocol of no sedation for critically ill patients receiving mechanical ventilation: a randomised trial. Lancet 2010;375(9713): 475–80.
28. Girard TD, Kress JP, Fuchs BD, et al. Efficacy and safety of a paired sedation and ventilator weaning protocol for mechanically ventilated patients in intensive care (awakening and breathing controlled trial): a randomised controlled trial. Lancet 2008;371(9607):126–34.
29. Brower RG. Consequences of bed rest. Crit Care Med 2009;37(Suppl 10): S422–8.
30. Herridge MS, Tansey CM, Matte A, et al. Functional disability 5 years after acute respiratory distress syndrome. N Engl J Med 2011;364(14):1293–304.
31. Ochala J, Gustafson AM, Diez ML, et al. Preferential skeletal muscle myosin loss in response to mechanical silencing in a novel rat intensive care unit model: underlying mechanisms. J Physiol 2011;589(Pt 8):2007–26.
32. Ibebunjo C, Martyn JA. Fiber atrophy, but not changes in acetylcholine receptor expression, contributes to the muscle dysfunction after immobilization. Crit Care Med 1999;27(2):275–85.
33. Kress JP, Pohlman AS, O'Connor MF, et al. Daily interruption of sedative infusions in critically ill patients undergoing mechanical ventilation. N Engl J Med 2000; 342(20):1471–7.

34. Brook AD, Ahrens TS, Schaiff R, et al. Effect of a nursing-implemented sedation protocol on the duration of mechanical ventilation. Crit Care Med 1999;27(12): 2609–15.
35. De Jonghe B, Bastuji-Garin S, Fangio P, et al. Sedation algorithm in critically ill patients without acute brain injury. Crit Care Med 2005;33(1):120–7.
36. Bailey P, Thomsen GE, Spuhler VJ, et al. Early activity is feasible and safe in respiratory failure patients. Crit Care Med 2007;35(1):139–45.
37. Morris PE, Goad A, Thompson C, et al. Early intensive care unit mobility therapy in the treatment of acute respiratory failure. Crit Care Med 2008;36(8):2238–43.
38. Morris PE, Griffin L, Berry M, et al. Receiving early mobility during an intensive care unit admission is a predictor of improved outcomes in acute respiratory failure. Am J Med Sci 2011;341(5):373–7.
39. Burtin C, Clerckx B, Robbeets C, et al. Early exercise in critically ill patients enhances short-term functional recovery. Crit Care Med 2009;37(9):2499–505.
40. Bourdin G, Barbier J, Burle JF, et al. The feasibility of early physical activity in intensive care unit patients: a prospective observational one-center study. Respir Care 2010;55(4):400–7.
41. Schweickert WD, Pohlman MC, Pohlman AS, et al. Early physical and occupational therapy in mechanically ventilated, critically ill patients: a randomised controlled trial. Lancet 2009;373(9678):1874–82.
42. Levine S, Nguyen T, Taylor N, et al. Rapid disuse atrophy of diaphragm fibers in mechanically ventilated humans. N Engl J Med 2008;358(13):1327–35.
43. Powers SK, Shanely RA, Coombes JS, et al. Mechanical ventilation results in progressive contractile dysfunction in the diaphragm. J Appl Phys 2002;92(5):1851–8.
44. Hussain SN, Mofarrahi M, Sigala I, et al. Mechanical ventilation-induced diaphragm disuse in humans triggers autophagy. Am J Respir Crit Care Med 2010;182(11):1377–86.
45. Ely EW, Baker AM, Dunagan DP, et al. Effect on the duration of mechanical ventilation of identifying patients capable of breathing spontaneously. N Engl J Med 1996;335(25):1864–9.
46. van den Berghe G, Wouters P, Weekers F, et al. Intensive insulin therapy in the critically ill patients. N Engl J Med 2001;345(19):1359–67.
47. Gosselink R, Bott J, Johnson M, et al. Physiotherapy for adult patients with critical illness: recommendations of the European respiratory society and European society of intensive care medicine task force on physiotherapy for critically ill patients. Intensive Care Med 2008;34(7):1188–99.
48. Hodgin KE, Nordon-Craft A, McFann KK, et al. Physical therapy utilization in intensive care units: results from a national survey. Crit Care Med 2009;37(2): 561–6 [Quiz: 6–8].
49. Martin UJ, Hincapie L, Nimchuk M, et al. Impact of whole-body rehabilitation in patients receiving chronic mechanical ventilation. Crit Care Med 2005;33(10): 2259–65.
50. Pohlman MC, Schweickert WD, Pohlman AS, et al. Feasibility of physical and occupational therapy beginning from initiation of mechanical ventilation. Crit Care Med 2010;38(11):2089–94.
51. Needham DM, Korupolu R, Zanni JM, et al. Early physical medicine and rehabilitation for patients with acute respiratory failure: a quality improvement project. Arch Phys Med Rehabil 2010;91(4):536–42.
52. Kho ME, Damluji A, Zanni JM, et al. Feasibility and observed safety of interactive video games for physical rehabilitation in the intensive care unit: a case series. J Crit Care 2012;27(2):219.e1–6.

Improving Intensive Care Unit Quality Using Collaborative Networks

Sam R. Watson, MSA, MA, CPPS[a], Damon C. Scales, MD, PhD[b,c,*]

KEYWORDS

• Quality improvement • Cooperative behavior • Collaboration • Cost-effectiveness
• Patient safety • Critical care • Intensive care units • Health economics

KEY POINTS

- Collaborative intensive care unit networks have successfully improved quality across entire health systems.
- These collaborative networks offer several advantages that include targeting a large number of patients, sharing of resources between sites, and implementing common measurement systems that can be used for audit and feedback or benchmarking.
- More research is needed to understand the mechanisms through which collaboratives lead to improved care delivery, and to demonstrate their cost-effectiveness in comparison with other approaches to system-level quality improvement.

INTRODUCTION

Critically ill patients require intensive monitoring and costly treatments. Despite advances, however, mortality remains high. Unfortunately, delays often exist in the publication and subsequent adoption of evidence-based practices. These delays may contribute to morbidity and mortality, and waste resources.[1–3] It is therefore vital that such errors of omission are avoided in these patients, and that evidence-based treatment is provided in a timely manner.

The challenge to the adoption of evidence-based best practice is twofold. First, the effort necessary to cull the evidence, identify valid measures, and implement change

---

Financial disclosure: There was no funding source for this article. D.C.S. is supported by a New Investigator Award from the Canadian Institutes for Health Research.

[a] Michigan Health Association Keystone Centre, 6215 West St. Joseph Highway, Lansing, MI 48917, USA; [b] Interdepartmental Division of Critical Care, University of Toronto, Toronto, Ontario, Canada; [c] Department of Critical Care Medicine, Sunnybrook Health Sciences Centre, 2075 Bayview Avenue, Room D108, Toronto, ON M4N 3M5, Canada
* Corresponding author. Department of Critical Care Medicine, Sunnybrook Health Sciences Centre, 2075 Bayview Avenue, Room D108, Toronto, ON M4N 3M5, Canada.
E-mail address: damon.scales@sunnybrook.ca

Crit Care Clin 29 (2013) 77–89
http://dx.doi.org/10.1016/j.ccc.2012.10.008 **criticalcare.theclinics.com**
0749-0704/13/$ – see front matter

can be significant, and in some cases may exceed the resources and abilities of individual clinicians. Second, implementing evidence-based therapies often requires that the behavior of clinicians be modified, and this requires effective strategies and often considerable time and effort.[4]

In addition, there is a need to expedite the rate of quality improvement. The recent report from the Institute of Medicine, *Best Care at Lower Cost: The Path to Continuously Learning Health Care in America*, emphasized that there have been limited gains in the improvement of quality and reduction of costs in health care, and highlighted the need to increase the scale of improvement efforts.[5] These challenges have motivated clinicians, researchers, and policy makers to promote larger statewide or regional quality-improvement campaigns over single-center quality initiatives.

There are many potential advantages to organizing health care centers to deliver system-level interventions to improve quality.[6] Most obviously, such approaches are appealing to health care funding bodies because more patients can benefit from the quality-improvement initiatives. Resources for quality improvement can be shared across sites, and there may be opportunities to share successful strategies and learning. Finally, accepted care practices can be standardized and common measurement systems can be implemented, allowing for benchmarking across centers.

Many systems and structures have been proposed to improve intensive care unit (ICU) quality across a system, for example, using telemedicine,[7] public reporting of quality measures, or creating reward-based or penalty-based pay-for-performance (P4P) schemes.[8,9] This article discusses the advantages and limitations of forming collaborative networks of hospitals, which link institutions together with the aim of improving quality across a system. Strategies that the authors consider important for ensuring the success of these networks are outlined, and the importance of ongoing evaluation to ensure that these networks achieve sustained impact and are cost-effective are discussed. The article concludes with a review of areas perceived to be important for future research.

WHAT IS AN ICU COLLABORATIVE NETWORK?

A collaborative network consists of multiple teams located in health care facilities in different geographic areas, or in different units within the same organization, working together to solve a practice gap.[10] Quality-improvement initiatives that involve more than one center are appealing for several reasons, in particular because the sharing of information and resources should create efficiencies while eliminating redundancies. The proposed advantage of the collaborative approach is predicated on the idea that learning from the successes of others and sharing of information between institutions or teams is more likely to lead to improvements in care through a group effort.[11–13] In other words, a collaborative network of hospitals or units working together would be expected to achieve better outcomes and faster results in quality-improvement initiatives than if they were working on the same initiatives alone.[14] In the last decade there have been several of these large-scale collaborative networks in the critical care environment, many claiming highly successful results.[15,16]

EXAMPLES IN CRITICAL CARE

A search was made of the available literature to identify collaborative networks that have been used to improve quality of care in ICUs. To identify potential publications, OVID Medline from 1996 to October 2012 was searched using the keyword "collaborative" combined with the medical subject headings "Critical Care" (243 citations) or "Intensive Care Units" (288 citations). From these, 17 publications describing multicentered collaborative networks targeting quality improvement in adult or pediatric ICUs were identified (**Table 1**). The number of centers involved ranged from 5 to 114. The most commonly used methods of dissemination were face-to-face workshops and teleconferences. A wide range of clinical practices were targeted by these collaborative networks, although the most frequently tackled problems were prevention of catheter-related bloodstream infections and ventilator-associated pneumonia (VAP).

Arguably the most well-known example of an ICU collaborative network is the Michigan Health and Hospital Association (MHA) Keystone Center's Keystone ICU project, in which the participants in the collaborative received standardized information on interventions and collected data using standard measures.[16] In addition, they addressed teamwork and patient-safety climate. Through face-to-face meetings and regular teleconferences, the ICU teams were able to learn collectively and share their individual experiences in the implementation of the interventions. Institutional performance data were shared anonymously, allowing the local ICU to compare itself against the entire collaborative.[17] The initiative involved more than 120 ICUs from around the state of Michigan, as well as 5 out-of-state ICUs. Of note, the collaborative linked the application of evidence-based medical interventions with the socioadaptive framework of improving teamwork and patient-safety culture. It focused on reducing 2 hospital-associated infections, central line–associated bloodstream infections (CLABSI), and VAP.[16,18] The MHA Keystone network was able to achieve sustainable reductions in both of these preventable complications.[19]

Similarly, 23 ICUs in all 11 acute care hospitals in Rhode Island formed a collaborative network to reduce ICU-related complications.[20] This collaborative model was associated with statewide reductions in CLABSI and VAP. The Veterans Affairs Midwest Care Network also developed a collaborative network involving 9 hospitals, and targeted these same preventable infections; this approach led to improved adoption and decreased infection rates in 8 of these hospitals.[21] A similar approach has been reported in pediatric ICUs.[22]

These collaboratives have typically reported success by documenting sustained reductions in preventable complications over time, or increased adherence to targeted care practices. More recently, some collaboratives have used more rigorous evaluations that are less vulnerable to confounding attributable to secular trends, using, for example, cluster randomization or interrupted time series. The results of these evaluations have not always been consistent; some collaborative approaches have yielded modest gains, whereas others have failed to show benefit. In Ontario, Canada, a collaborative involving 15 community ICUs (the Ontario ICU Best Practices Project) achieved modest improvements in adherence to 6 quality-process measures, especially when baseline compliance was low.[23] A multifaceted intervention to improve end-of-life care that was delivered to 6 active hospitals did not lead to improved family-reported or nurse-reported quality of dying in comparison with 6 control hospitals.[24] These results have led to recommendations that the implementation of future collaborative networks should use more rigorous evaluations, especially considering that improvements in some of the more commonly targeted complications, for example CLABSI and VAP, have been observed over time in regions without active large-scale quality-improvement initiatives.[25,26]

ESSENTIAL ELEMENTS OF A COLLABORATIVE

Implementation science is a new and evolving field, with a paucity of research directed at understanding critical factors in the successful implementation of large-scale collaboratives.[25,27] However, from the experience of the Keystone ICU project and

Table 1
Characteristics of critical care collaborative networks

Collaborative	Number of Centers Participating	Geography of Collaborative	Key Interventions	Methods of Dissemination (Face-to-Face Workshops, Teleconference, etc)
The Canadian ICU Collaborative[39,40]	50	National (Canada)	1. Transfusions 2. Ventilator-associated pneumonia prevention 3. High-risk medications 4. Sepsis 5. Cardiac arrests 6. Central line–associated bloodstream infection prevention	Face-to-face workshops Teleconference
On The CUSP: STOP BSI, Hawaii[41]	16	State/Provincial (Hawaii, USA)	Central line–associated bloodstream infection prevention	Face-to-face workshops Web content Teleconference
Vermont Oxford Network: promotion of evidence based surfactant treatment for preterm infants of 23–29 wk gestation[42]	114	National (USA)	Evidence-based surfactant treatment for preterm infants of 23–29 wk gestation	Face-to-face workshops Web content Teleconference
Vermont Oxford Network[43]	10	National (USA)	1. Nosocomial infection 2. Chronic lung disease	Face-to-face workshops
Network-Based Pilot Program to Improve Palliative Care in the Intensive Care Unit[44]	5	Regional (New York/New Jersey, USA VA hospitals)	1. Identify family's cardiopulmonary resuscitation preference 2. Offer the patient and family social work support and spiritual support 3. Conduct an interdisciplinary family meeting to discuss the patient's and/or family diagnosis, prognosis, goals of care	Face-to-face workshops Teleconference

The Ohio Perinatal Quality Collaborative[45]	20	State/Provincial (Ohio, USA)	1. Promotion of ultrasound confirmation of gestational age <20 wk 2. Promotion and adoption of American College of Obstetricians and Gynecologists schedule 3. Birth criteria 4. Dating criteria optimal 5. Specific indication for scheduled birth 6. Documented discussion of risks and benefits of scheduled birth 7. Improved obstetric-pediatric communication 8. Culture of safety	Face-to-face workshops Teleconference
Keystone ICU[16]	72	State/Provincial (Michigan, USA)	1. Central line–associated bloodstream infection prevention 2. Ventilator-associated pneumonia prevention 3. Comprehensive unit-based safety program	Face-to-face workshops Web content Teleconference
Integrating a multidisciplinary mobility program into intensive care practice[46]	8	National (USA)	Progressive mobility	Face-to-face workshops Toolkits Teleconference
Neonatal Intensive Care Quality Improvement Collaborative 2000: ALI[47]	9	National (USA)	1. Vitamin A supplementation 2. Decrease fluid administration 3. Postextubation CPAP 4. Permissive hypercarbia 5. Decrease dexamethasone 6. Prophylactic surfactant delivery room NCPAP 7. High-frequency ventilation or low-VT ventilation 8. Gentle ventilation in the delivery room	Face-to-face workshops Web content Teleconference Site visits

(*continued on next page*)

Table 1
(continued)

Collaborative	Number of Centers Participating	Geography of Collaborative	Key Interventions	Methods of Dissemination (Face-to-Face Workshops, Teleconference, etc)
Vermont Oxford Neonatal Evidence-Based Quality Improvement Collaborative[48]	6	National (USA)	Nosocomial infection prevention	Face-to-face workshops Teleconference
A statewide quality-improvement collaborative to reduce neonatal central line–associated bloodstream infections[49]	13	State/Provincial (California, USA)	Central line–associated bloodstream infection prevention	Face-to-face workshops Web content Teleconference Site visits
The Ontario ICU Clinical Best Practices Project[23]	15	State/Provincial (Ontario, Canada)	1. Prevention of ventilator-associated pneumonia 2. Prophylaxis against deep vein thrombosis 3. Daily spontaneous breathing trials 4. Prevention of catheter-related bloodstream infections 5. Early enteral feeding Initiation of enteral feeds within 48 h of ICU admission 6. Decubitus ulcer prevention	Video conference Web content Annual face-to-face workshops

Child Health Corporation of America multicenter collaborative[50]	20	National (USA)	1. Prevention practices (eg, SBAR and mock codes) 2. Detection practices (eg, pediatric early warning system) 3. Correction practices (eg, algorithms for shock, respiratory distress, neurologic changes)	Face-to-face workshops Web content Teleconference
Child Health Corporation of America multicenter collaborative[22]	26	National (USA)	Central line–associated bloodstream infection prevention	Face-to-face workshops Web content Teleconference
The Rhode Island ICU Collaborative[51]	11	State/Provincial (Rhode Island, USA)	1. Central line–associated bloodstream infection prevention 2. Ventilator-associated pneumonia prevention 3. Comprehensive unit-based safety program	Face-to-face workshops Web content Teleconference
A statewide collaborative to decrease NICU central line–associated bloodstream infections[52]	19	State/Provincial (New York, USA)	Central line–associated bloodstream infection prevention	Face-to-face workshops
A collaborative to reduce ventilator-associated pneumonia in Thailand[53]	18	National (Thailand)	Ventilator-associated pneumonia prevention	National and regional face-to-face workshops

Abbreviations: CPAP, continuous positive airway pressure; ICU, intensive care unit; NCPAP, nasal CPAP; NICU, neonatal ICU; SBAR, Situation/Background/Assessment/Recommendation; VA, Veterans Administration; VT, tidal volume.

the Ontario ICU Best Practices Project, there are several essential elements that contribute to the success and sustainability of these networks.

First, tasking a central body with summarizing the available evidence and identifying the interventions that are most likely to result in a change in clinician behavior reduces the burden on individual facilities and busy clinicians.[4] The synthesis of evidence into a useful and practical intervention can be resource intensive, and in many cases may exceed the capability of many hospitals, especially nonacademic facilities.

Second, developing a limited set of standardized measures that are linked to the intervention and desired outcome is a critical aspect of the collaborative process. Without credible measures, clinicians are less likely to believe that the interventions are effective. Furthermore, choosing measures that can be directly linked to the targeted practices ensures that participants can associate their efforts with meaningful improvements. Focusing on only a limited (rather than exhaustive) set of valid measures helps to limit the resources that are required for data collection; if data-collection efforts become overly burdensome, this can detract from the intended focus of the collaborative.

Third, a successful collaborative will engage frontline clinicians and address quality targets that are clinically important and relevant. Ensuring that participating ICUs have an opportunity to provide input and contribute to the overall approach that is adopted will increase the likelihood of buy-in; if an intervention is perceived to have limited value to the physicians involved, they are less likely to participate or be supportive. Some collaboratives have engaged frontline clinicians with face-to-face educational sessions, whereas others have used telemedicine; the comparative effectiveness of each should be a topic of future research.

Developing partnerships with payers can also create advantages. For example, in Michigan the largest commercial payer began to include the Keystone ICU project in its P4P incentive, and this added additional incentives to participation. The Blue Cross Blue Shield of Michigan (BCBSM) first provided financial incentives to hospitals in the collaborative that submitted data. This incentive encouraged those organizations that may have been less likely to participate to report data on a regular basis. The incentive was subsequently switched from a pay-for-participation to a P4P scheme, in which hospitals were rewarded only when there was improved adoption of processes that were linked to the outcomes.

Centralized support for the collection and reporting of data is a core element of a collaborative quality-improvement initiative. A system of audit and feedback helps to maintain the credibility of the intervention and monitor its ongoing effectiveness, and to convince stakeholders that resources could not be better directed elsewhere. In Michigan, data submitted to the project management team were reported back within a 6-week time frame. The rapid reporting of the ICUs' performance, along with a comparison with other ICUs in the project, provided timely feedback to the frontline teams and was perceived to be important for maintaining engagement. Similarly, in the Ontario ICU quality-improvement collaborative, timely audit-feedback of comparative performance information was cited by participants as being the most important driver of change through "friendly competition." Furthermore, the comparisons with other participating ICUs were deemed to increase communication within ICUs and elicit support from hospital leadership.[23,28]

The optimal size, geography, and scope of a large-scale collaborative remain unknown. State-level or other regionalization may offer some advantages (eg, fostering healthy competition between sites) that may be difficult to achieve with much larger initiatives such as the Institute for Healthcare Improvement 100,000 Lives Campaign.[29] Such competition has been found to be a key element contributing to the success of some collaboratives.[28]

Finally, the collaborative network cannot focus solely on the clinical processes and outcomes. It must have a component that actually addresses changing the behavior of clinicians. Collectively these behaviors, referred to as the ICU's culture, are influenced by the perspectives and attitudes of the clinical staff toward patient safety and teamwork. In the Keystone ICU project, the application of interventions that specifically addressed how teams worked together to solve problems, prevent harm, and communicate with each other were applied alongside the technical interventions to prevent CLABSI and VAP. The use of tools to foster and develop teamwork, such as daily goals and "learning from defects," were used to foster an environment where physicians and nurses, as well as other members of the care team, respected the input of each other in the provision of care.[30–32] There is much emerging literature demonstrating that improved teamwork and safety culture lead to better outcomes for patients.[33,34]

EVALUATING BENEFITS AND UNINTENDED CONSEQUENCES

The authors believe that more research is needed to evaluate the effectiveness of ICU collaborative networks, and also to better understand which factors contribute to their success or failure. To date, most large-scale quality-improvement interventions including collaboratives have been evaluated using the before-after study design or analyses of administrative data. Although these offer advantages because they are simple and feasible, they can be vulnerable to confounding even when sophisticated time-series analyses are used.[35,36] Collaboratives are increasingly being studied using more rigorous study designs, for example, cluster randomized trials[23]; these approaches can help account for temporal trends that may have been unrelated to the intervention.[25] A challenge in cluster randomized trials for studying collaboratives is that they require some hospitals to receive no intervention if randomized to a control arm. The Ontario collaborative overcame this challenge by using an "active control group," so that each group of ICUs received the active behavior-change intervention targeting one care practice and simultaneously acted as a control group for the other group of ICUs that received the active behavior-change intervention targeting a different care practice. Stepped-wedge randomization is another approach to evaluating large-scale quality-improvement initiatives that is becoming increasingly used to evaluate collaborative networks.[37,38] This study design involves randomizing groups to receive the intervention at different time points and in sequence; groups that have not yet received the intervention remain as "controls" until a time point that is predefined by the randomization scheme. This approach has appeal because it ensures that all groups will receive the quality-improvement intervention by the end of the evaluation, and can make the roll-out more manageable. However, as with cluster randomized trials, a disadvantage is that many hospitals will not be part of the collaborative at the start of the implementation.

FUTURE RESEARCH

The success of collaborative projects such as the Keystone ICU project has compelled many regions and jurisdictions to consider similar large-scale quality-improvement initiatives. However, much remains to be learned about the effectiveness of these collaboratives and their mechanisms of action. For example, what makes some collaborative networks more effective than others? Are some care practices and behaviors more amenable to change using collaboratives? Are these collaborative networks cost-effective, especially compared with multiple single-unit quality-improvement initiatives or other approaches to improving care across a system? These and other questions outlined in **Box 1** highlight the many knowledge gaps

Box 1
Questions for future research involving ICU collaborative networks

Research on the Effectiveness of Collaborative Networks

What makes some collaborative networks more effective than others?

How sustainable are the improvements that can be achieved using collaborative networks?

Are collaborative networks cost-effective compared with multiple single-unit quality-improvement initiatives, and in comparison with other system-level quality-improvement initiatives (eg, public reporting or P4P)?

Research on How Collaborative Networks Change Behavior

Are some care practices and behaviors more amenable to change using collaborative networks?

What components of a quality-improvement intervention are most suited to use in a collaborative network (eg, education, reminders, audit-feedback, and so forth)?

Does competition versus cooperation lead to more effective uptake and adoption, and foster change in behavior?

How much contact is required between frontline clinicians and the coordinating center, or project leaders?

Which members of the health care team and/or administration need to be involved to make a collaborative most successful?

What improvement knowledge do frontline providers engaged in the project need?

Can telemedicine connections between geographically separated ICUs achieve the same degree of motivation among participants as face-to-face meetings?

that persist. There are great opportunities for further research to explore these issues and to ensure that these collaborative networks, which typically involve many hospitals, clinicians, and resources, can achieve their goals of improving system-level quality and becoming cost-effective.

SUMMARY

Collaborative ICU networks have successfully improved quality across entire health systems. These networks offer several advantages that include targeting a large number of patients, sharing of resources between sites, and implementing common measurement systems that can be used for audit and feedback or benchmarking. More research is needed to understand the mechanisms through which collaboratives lead to improved delivery of care and to demonstrate their cost-effectiveness in comparison with other approaches to system-level quality improvement.

REFERENCES

1. Kohn L, Corrigan J, Donaldson M. To err is human: building a safer health system. Washington, DC: National Academy Press; 2000.
2. McGlynn EA, Asch SM, Adams J, et al. The quality of health care delivered to adults in the United States. N Engl J Med 2003;348(26):2635–45.
3. Institute of Medicine. Crossing the quality chasm: a new health system for the 21st century. Washington, DC: National Academy Press; 2001.
4. Pronovost PJ, Berenholtz SM, Needham DM. Translating evidence into practice: a model for large scale knowledge translation. BMJ 2008;337:a1714.

5. Committee on the Learning Healthcare System in America. Best care at lower cost: the path to continuously learning health care in America. Institute of Medicine. Washington, DC: National Academies Press; 2012.
6. Scales D. Partnering with health care payers to advance the science of quality improvement: lessons from the field. Am J Respir Crit Care Med 2011;184:987–8.
7. Lilly CM, Cody S, Zhao H, et al. Hospital mortality, length of stay, and preventable complications among critically ill patients before and after tele-ICU reengineering of critical care processes. JAMA 2011;305(21):2175–83.
8. Kahn JM, Scales DC, Au DH, et al. An official American Thoracic Society policy statement: pay-for-performance in pulmonary, critical care, and sleep medicine. Am J Respir Crit Care Med 2010;181(7):752–61.
9. Khanduja K, Scales DC, Adhikari NK. Pay for performance in the intensive care unit—opportunity or threat? Crit Care Med 2009;37(3):852–8.
10. Schouten LM, Hulscher ME, van Everdingen JJ, et al. Evidence for the impact of quality improvement collaboratives: systematic review. BMJ 2008;336(7659): 1491–4.
11. IHI Innovation White Paper. The breakthrough series: IHI's collaborative model for achieving breakthrough improvement. Boston: Institute for Health Improvement; 2003.
12. Leatherman S. Optimizing quality collaboratives. Qual Saf Health Care 2002; 11(4):307.
13. Berwick DM. Continuous improvement as an ideal in health care. N Engl J Med 1989;320(1):53–6.
14. Huxham C, Macdonald D. Introducing collaborative advantage: achieving inter-organizational effectiveness through meta-strategy. Manag Decis 1992;30(3):50–6.
15. Ferrer R, Artigas A, Levy MM, et al. Improvement in process of care and outcome after a multicenter severe sepsis educational program in Spain. JAMA 2008; 299(19):2294–303.
16. Pronovost P, Needham D, Berenholtz S, et al. An intervention to decrease catheter-related bloodstream infections in the ICU. N Engl J Med 2006;355(26): 2725–32.
17. Dixon-Woods M, Bosk CL, Aveling EL, et al. Explaining Michigan: developing an ex post theory of a quality improvement program. Milbank Q 2011;89(2):167–205.
18. Pronovost PJ, Goeschel CA, Colantuoni E, et al. Sustaining reductions in catheter related bloodstream infections in Michigan intensive care units: observational study. BMJ 2010;340:c309.
19. Berenholtz SM, Pham JC, Thompson DA, et al. Collaborative cohort study of an intervention to reduce ventilator-associated pneumonia in the intensive care unit. Infect Control Hosp Epidemiol 2011;32(4):305–14.
20. McNicoll L, DePalo VA, Cornell M, et al. The Rhode Island ICU Collaborative: the first statewide collaborative four years later. Med Health R I 2009;92(8):272–3, 276.
21. Bonello RS, Fletcher CE, Becker WK, et al. An intensive care unit quality improvement collaborative in nine Department of Veterans Affairs hospitals: reducing ventilator-associated pneumonia and catheter-related bloodstream infection rates. Jt Comm J Qual Patient Saf 2008;34(11):639–45.
22. Jeffries HE, Mason W, Brewer M, et al. Prevention of central venous catheter-associated bloodstream infections in pediatric intensive care units: a performance improvement collaborative. Infect Control Hosp Epidemiol 2009;30(7):645–51.
23. Scales DC, Dainty K, Hales B, et al. A multifaceted intervention for quality improvement in a network of intensive care units: a cluster randomized trial. JAMA 2011;305(4):363–72.

24. Curtis JR, Nielsen EL, Treece PD, et al. Effect of a quality-improvement intervention on end-of-life care in the intensive care unit: a randomized trial. Am J Respir Crit Care Med 2011;183(3):348–55.
25. Curtis JR, Levy MM. Improving the science and politics of quality improvement. JAMA 2011;305(4):406–7.
26. Zuschneid I, Schwab F, Geffers C, et al. Reducing central venous catheter-associated primary bloodstream infections in intensive care units is possible: data from the German nosocomial infection surveillance system. Infect Control Hosp Epidemiol 2003;24(7):501–5.
27. White DE, Straus SE, Stelfox HT, et al. What is the value and impact of quality and safety teams? A scoping review. Implement Sci 2011;6:97.
28. Dainty KN, Scales DC, Sinuff T, et al. Competition in collaborative clothing: a qualitative case study of influences on collaborative quality improvement in ICU. BMJ Qual Saf 2012, in press.
29. Berwick DM, Calkins DR, McCannon CJ, et al. The 100,000 lives campaign: setting a goal and a deadline for improving health care quality. JAMA 2006; 295(3):324–7.
30. Schwartz JM, Nelson KL, Saliski M, et al. The daily goals communication sheet: a simple and novel tool for improved communication and care. Jt Comm J Qual Patient Saf 2008;34(10):608–13, 561.
31. Berenholtz SM, Hartsell TL, Pronovost PJ. Learning from defects to enhance morbidity and mortality conferences. Am J Med Qual 2009;24(3):192–5.
32. Pronovost PJ, Holzmueller CG, Martinez E, et al. A practical tool to learn from defects in patient care. Jt Comm J Qual Patient Saf 2006;32(2):102–8.
33. Jain M, Miller L, Belt D, et al. Decline in ICU adverse events, nosocomial infections and cost through a quality improvement initiative focusing on teamwork and culture change. Qual Saf Health Care 2006;15(4):235–9.
34. Waters HR, Korn R Jr, Colantuoni E, et al. The business case for quality: economic analysis of the Michigan Keystone Patient Safety Program in ICUs. Am J Med Qual 2011;26(5):333–9.
35. Eccles M, Grimshaw J, Campbell M, et al. Research designs for studies evaluating the effectiveness of change and improvement strategies. Qual Saf Health Care 2003;12(1):47–52.
36. Fan E, Laupacis A, Pronovost PJ, et al. How to use an article about quality improvement. JAMA 2010;304(20):2279–87.
37. Dainty KN, Scales DC, Brooks SC, et al. A knowledge translation collaborative to improve the use of therapeutic hypothermia in post-cardiac arrest patients: protocol for a stepped wedge randomized trial. Implement Sci 2011;6:4.
38. Hussey MA, Hughes JP. Design and analysis of stepped wedge cluster randomized trials. Contemp Clin Trials 2007;28(2):182–91.
39. Mawdsley C, Northway T. The Canadian ICU collaborative to improve patient safety in the ICU: accelerating best practice to the bedside. Dynamics 2006; 17(3):26–7.
40. Northway T, Mawdsley C. The Canadian ICU collaborative: working together to improve patient outcomes as an interprofessional team. Dynamics 2008;19(1): 30–1.
41. Lin DM, Weeks K, Bauer L, et al. Eradicating central line-associated bloodstream infections statewide: the Hawaii experience. Am J Med Qual 2012;27(2):124–9.
42. Horbar JD, Carpenter JH, Buzas J, et al. Collaborative quality improvement to promote evidence based surfactant for preterm infants: a cluster randomised trial. BMJ 2004;329(7473):1004.

43. Horbar JD, Rogowski J, Plsek PE, et al. Collaborative quality improvement for neonatal intensive care. NIC/Q Project Investigators of the Vermont Oxford Network. Pediatrics 2001;107(1):14–22.
44. Penrod JD, Luhrs CA, Livote EE, et al. Implementation and evaluation of a network-based pilot program to improve palliative care in the intensive care unit. J Pain Symptom Manage 2011;42(5):668–71.
45. Donovan EF, Lannon C, Bailit J, et al. A statewide initiative to reduce inappropriate scheduled births at 36(0/7)-38(6/7) weeks' gestation. Am J Obstet Gynecol 2010;202(3):243–8.
46. Bassett RD, Vollman KM, Brandwene L, et al. Integrating a multidisciplinary mobility programme into intensive care practice (IMMPTP): a multicentre collaborative. Intensive Crit Care Nurs 2012;28(2):88–97.
47. Sharek PJ, Baker R, Litman F, et al. Evaluation and development of potentially better practices to prevent chronic lung disease and reduce lung injury in neonates. Pediatrics 2003;111(4 Pt 2):e426–31.
48. Kilbride HW, Powers R, Wirtschafter DD, et al. Evaluation and development of potentially better practices to prevent neonatal nosocomial bacteremia. Pediatrics 2003;111(4 Pt 2):e504–18.
49. Wirtschafter DD, Pettit J, Kurtin P, et al. A statewide quality improvement collaborative to reduce neonatal central line-associated blood stream infections. J Perinatol 2010;30(3):170–81.
50. Hayes LW, Dobyns EL, DiGiovine B, et al. A multicenter collaborative approach to reducing pediatric codes outside the ICU. Pediatrics 2012;129(3):e785–91.
51. DePalo VA, McNicoll L, Cornell M, et al. The Rhode Island ICU collaborative: a model for reducing central line-associated bloodstream infection and ventilator-associated pneumonia statewide. Qual Saf Health Care 2010;19(6): 555–61.
52. Schulman J, Stricof RL, Stevens TP, et al. Development of a statewide collaborative to decrease NICU central line-associated bloodstream infections. J Perinatol 2009;29(9):591–9.
53. Unahalekhaka A, Jamulitrat S, Chongsuvivatwong V, et al. Using a collaborative to reduce ventilator-associated pneumonia in Thailand. Jt Comm J Qual Patient Saf 2007;33(7):387–94.

Does Value-Based Purchasing Enhance Quality of Care and Patient Outcomes in the ICU?

James M. O'Brien Jr, MD, MSc[a,*], Anupam Kumar, MD[b], Mark L. Metersky, MD[c]

KEYWORDS

- Value-based purchasing • Pay for performance • Health care reform
- Quality improvement • Health care quality

KEY POINTS

- Reimbursement for health care is moving from one based on volume of services to one based on quality of care, called value-based purchasing (VBP).
- The National Quality Forum (NQF) and the Centers for Medicare and Medicaid Services (CMS) are influential in the development of the infrastructure and execution of VBP.
- Critical care services are likely targets for VBP due to the expense of the provided care and variation in processes and outcomes from care.
- There is little existing evidence that VBP will improve the quality of care in the ICU or elsewhere in the health care continuum.
- The effectiveness of VBP on improving quality of care and patient outcomes will be determined after its implementation.

INTRODUCTION

The CMS reports that health care expenditures grew 3.9% in 2010, with total health expenditures reaching $2.6 trillion, or 17.9% of the nation's gross domestic product.[1] The two largest consumers of health care dollars in 2010 were hospital care ($814.0 billion) and physician and clinical services ($515.5 billion), which comprised more than half of all health care dollars spent. Because the federal government finances the greatest portion of total health spending (29%), Congress has focused efforts to curb health care expenditures. A major effort is to migrate from a paradigm in which reimbursement is driven by the quantity of services provided to reimbursement based

[a] Quality and Patient Safety, Riverside Methodist Hospital, 3535 Olentangy River Road, 5 Blue – 5135E, Columbus, OH 43214, USA; [b] Department of Medicine, Hartford Hospital, University of Connecticut Health Center, 263 Farmington Avenue, Farmington, CT 06030-1321, USA; [c] Division of Pulmonary and Critical Care Medicine, University of Connecticut Health Center, 263 Farmington Avenue, Farmington, CT 06030-1321, USA
* Corresponding author.
E-mail address: Jobrien4@ohiohealth.com

Crit Care Clin 29 (2013) 91–112
http://dx.doi.org/10.1016/j.ccc.2012.10.002 criticalcare.theclinics.com
0749-0704/13/$ – see front matter

on the quality of care. One major initiative in this effort is the implementation of pay-for-performance programs, also known as VBP. Integral to VBP is the use of performance measures (PMs)—standard metrics by which a health care provider and/or facility is compared with their past performance and contemporary performance by others.

The ICU is a likely target for efforts toward improving value, due to expended costs and variation in care provided to critically ill patients. Estimates are that, despite accounting for only 10% of in-patient beds, care for patients in the ICU accounts for 13.7% of hospital expenses, 4.1% of national health expenses, and 0.66% of the gross domestic product.[2] Medicare beneficiaries account for 42% to 52% of ICU admissions[3,4] and 40% of Medicare beneficiaries receive care in an ICU during their terminal illness, consuming 25% of all Medicare expenditures.[5,6]

ICU patients have complex medical and surgical disease, often with multiorgan dysfunction. As a result, these patients are some of the most fragile, whose care requires collaboration of multiple disciplines and provides considerable opportunity for medical errors and harm.[7] The evidence base for improving the care of ICU patients continues to expand and includes lung-protective ventilation for acute lung injury[8]; rapid treatment of severe sepsis and septic shock with antibiotics[9]; avoidance of hospital-acquired infections, including central line–associated bloodstream infections (CLABSIs)[10] and ventilator-associated pneumonia[11]; and judicious use of sedatives with protocolized interruptions paired with assessments of readiness for extubation in mechanically ventilated patients.[12] Despite a growing evidence base, implementation of best practice has been incomplete and delayed.[9,13–15] The care of critically ill patients and their outcome from this care is a prime target of efforts to improve value because of the federal dollars consumed, variability in care and outcome, and growing evidence base.

The focus of this article is on exploring the history and future of VBP and examining the evidence that VBP affects quality in general and for critical care patients specifically. The motivation for VBP is to increase the value of health care—defined as quality produced per cost, or quality ÷ cost.[16] The ability of VBP to affect cost (which might affect value without affecting quality) is beyond this discussion but remains controversial.[17] Quality-improvement projects within practices and facilities and across collaboratives are addressed in both the article by Watson and Scales as well as the article by Tropello and colleagues in this issue. Although many organizations develop and endorse PMs and private health insurers are incorporating VBP into their strategy, this article focuses on PMs endorsed by the NQF and incorporated into the CMS VBP program, because this is the most influential and publicly available program for review. As of 2010, however, 96% of health plans had VBP programs in place or in development,[18] so this is likely to become a significant mechanism for health care reimbursement and the CMS strategy may prove a blueprint for other plans.

THE NATIONAL QUALITY FORUM AND PERFORMANCE MEASURES

The NQF was created as a result of a President's Advisory Commission on Consumer Protection and Quality in the Health Care Industry report to "implement a comprehensive plan for measuring health care quality and reporting the results of such measures to the public."[19] Because of this mission, the NQF has been at the center of the movement toward VBP. Enhancing its prominence, the Medicare Improvements and Extension Act of 2006 and the Tax Relief and Health Care Act of 2006 designated NQF as the responsible organization for the review, endorsement, and maintenance of national PMs.[20] As a result, before inclusion in CMS programs, a PM must first be endorsed by NQF. The NQF is governed by a 27-member board, including the directors of the Agency for Healthcare Research and Quality (AHRQ), the CMS, and the

National Institutes of Health and is comprised of membership councils representing multiple stakeholders in health care, including consumers, health plans, health professionals, industry, and other organizations.[21]

The NQF does not develop PMs per se. Instead, the NQF has an established process for the submission, review, and endorsement of PMs developed by measure stewards.[22] In general, this process begins with a call for measures. As a result of this request, measure stewards assume responsibility for the submission of a measure for potential endorsement to NQF. Common organizations serving as measure stewards include The Joint Commission, the CMS, the Physician Consortium for Performance Improvement, and medical specialty societies. Proposed PMs are reviewed by an NQF steering cmmittee and, as needed, a technical advisory panel. PMs are judged by NQF measure evaluation criteria (**Box 1**).[23] PMs passing initial review are released for public comment. This process may result in revision of the PM before voting by the NQF members. After this vote, the steering committee makes a recommendation to the NQF Consensus Standards Approval Committee, which makes a final recommendation to the NQF board of Directors to fully endorse the PM, endorse the PM for a limited time pending testing, or not endorse the PM. All PMs are reassessed every 3 years for continued endorsement or retirement.

Box 1
NQF criteria for performance measure evaluation

1. Importance to measure and report—measures must be judged to meet all 3 subcriteria to evaluate the PM further
   a. High impact—including addressing identified national priorities
   b. Performance gap—demonstration of quality problems and opportunity to improve
   c. Evidence to support the measure focus—rationale supports the relationship of health outcome to process or structure of care; evidence supports that the measure focus leads to a desired health outcome; measure is valued by patients; measures efficiency, combining resource use, and quality
2. Scientific acceptability—measures must be judged to meet both subcriteria to evaluate the PM further
   a. Reliability—measure is well-defined and precisely specified, allowing for comparability across organizations; measure data elements are repeatable
   b. Validity—measure specifications are consistent with the evidence to support the focus of measurement; measure data elements correctly reflect quality of care provided; exclusions are supported by clinical evidence; evidence-based risk-adjusting models are specified and incorporated; meaningful differences in performance can be determined; multiple data sources produce similar results
   c. Disparities—identified disparities are handled through stratification of results
3. Usability—demonstration that information produced is meaningful for public reporting and for informing quality improvement
4. Feasibility—data elements are routinely generated during clinical care; data elements are available in electronic health records (EHRs); a mechanism for auditing is available; data collection can be implemented
5. Comparison with related or competing measures—measure specifications are harmonized with related measures or the differences are specified; measure is superior to competing measures or multiple measures are justified

Data from National Quality Forum Measure Evaluation Criteria. National Quality Forum, Washington DC; 2011. Available at: http://www.qualityforum.org/docs/measure_evaluation_criteria.aspx.

After NQF endorsement, the PM is available publicly for use in VBP programs, maintenance of certification efforts, and various quality improvement projects. Therefore, NQF endorsement is a critical step in the adoption of a PM into VBP. For the CMS, NQF endorsement is required for a PM to be incorporated into its VBP program. Therefore, a review of currently endorsed NQF measures allows for a window into future targets for CMS efforts to improve quality and reduce cost. **Table 1** outlines selected NQF-endorsed PMs applicable to critical care. The roster of endorsed measures changes, however, with endorsement of new PMs and retirement of others. NQF supplies an on-line search of all approved PMs.[24]

CMS AND VALUE-BASED PURCHASING

Although the foundation for and initial efforts toward VBP preceded its enactment, the Patient Protection and Accountable Care Act of 2010 (also known as the Affordable Care Act [ACA]) required the specification of a hospital VBP program built on the Hospital Inpatient Quality Reporting Program. Foundational efforts included the exclusion of select hospital-acquired conditions (HACs) from upgrading of diagnosis-related group (DRG) due to complications and providing incentives for reporting data and implementing EHRs. The hospital VBP[25] in the ACA applies to approximately 3500 acute care hospitals and provides a mechanism for adjusting reimbursement based on quality.

The hospital VBP is required to be a budget-neutral proposal. Therefore, the CMS will fund the program by reducing the DRG payments on all Medicare discharges. Past performance results in withholding of funds for future patients. For example, PMs for care provided from July 1, 2011, to March 31, 2012, affects reimbursements for admissions starting on October 1, 2012. The at-risk pool is 1% of the DRG payment in fiscal year (FY) 2013 and will increase by 0.25% per year to a maximum of 2% in FY 2017. In determining performance, the CMS sets 2 targets: (1) the benchmark—set at the average performance of the top decile of hospitals during the baseline period, and (2) the threshold—set at the median performance score for all hospitals during the baseline period. Scoring is then based on points earned through performance in comparison with other hospitals (achievement points) or in comparison with the institution's baseline performance (improvement points). The higher of the 2 points is then awarded for that measure. The measure scores are totaled and normalized for each domain and domain scores are converted to a total performance score. This score is then translated into an incentive payment by a linear exchange function. Theoretically, hospitals can earn up to the maximum percentage withheld in the at-risk pool. In other words, with 1% at-risk in the FY 2013 pool, the range of incentives hospitals could receive extends from a 1% bonus to a 1% penalty on Medicare discharges.

Table 2 outlines the measures and relative weight of each domain for FYs 2013–2015 (FY 2015 is not finalized as of this writing). In FY 2013, this score was based on 12 clinical processes of care measures (comprising 70% of the score) and a patient experience score—the Hospital Consumer Assessment of Healthcare Providers and Systems survey (providing the remaining 30% of the score). The CMS has the authority to alter the measures and domains included from year to year. Measures must be selected from those reported under the Hospital Inpatient Quality Reporting Program program (and, therefore, endorsed by NQF) and be published on Hospital Compare (http://www.hospitalcompare.hhs.gov/) for at least 1 year before the start of the performance period. The CMS must provide notice of measures at least 60 days before the start of the performance period, usually as a proposed rule notification in the *Federal Register*. The CMS may also retire measures, generally if they believe that performance has been topped out and no further improvement can occur.

A second component of the effort to improve value among CMS beneficiaries specified in the ACA is the Hospital Readmission Reduction Program.[26] This program calculates the ratio of observed to expected readmissions within 30 days of discharge for Medicare discharges due to heart failure, acute myocardial infarction, and pneumonia, based on DRG claims. For FY 2013 (taking effect for claims after October 1, 2012), the period determining this adjustment was from July 1, 2008, to June 30, 2011. For this initiative, there is no opportunity for receiving additional reimbursement. Instead, a percentage of DRG reimbursement is withheld from future claims on all Medicare discharges—not just those DRGs targeted for reduction of readmissions. For FY 2013, the maximum penalty is 1%, with increases to 2% in FY 2014 and 3% in 2015. In FY 2015, the list of conditions targeted for readmission reduction efforts can be expanded to include other conditions, with chronic obstructive pulmonary disease and several cardiac and vascular surgical procedures likely candidates.

One of the earlier attempts by the CMS to affect value through reimbursement mechanisms was by declining payment for certain HACs.[27] As part of the Deficit Reduction Act of 2005, the CMS was to identify conditions that are high volume and/or cost that could have been reasonably prevented and with their occurrence resulted in the assignment of a case to a DRG with a higher payment when that HAC was present as a secondary diagnosis. Starting on October 1, 2008, hospitals were paid as if the HAC never occurred, rather than receiving additional payment, unless the HAC was present on admission to that hospital. **Box 2** outlines the HACs included in the FY 2013 CMS final rule.

The Physician Quality Reporting System (PQRS) is a VBP program tied to individual provider performance.[28] Initial reporting began in 2007 and any physician seeing Medicare patients is allowed to participate. Participants have an option of choosing 3 or more relevant quality measures (among 208 available measures and 22 measure groups for 2012) to be reported as category II Current Procedural Terminology (CPT) codes, through an approved registry, through an EHR, or through maintenance of certification programs. **Table 3** highlights PQRS measures potentially relevant to critical care practitioners.

Initially, physicians received bonus payments for reporting performance or nonperformance of these measures—not how often they provided the recommended care. In 2012, participants could earn a 0.5% incentive (down from 2% in 2010) for reporting data on 3 measures for at least 50% of qualifying Medicare encounters or by reporting on a single measure group for 30 qualifying encounters. This adjustment in reimbursement applies to all Medicare claims, not only those with reported measures. Beginning in 2015, there will not be an incentive for reporting but a penalty of 1.5% for physicians who elect not to participate or are found unsuccessful (report on <50% of eligible encounters). Again, this applies to all Medicare encounters for that practitioner. The determination of this penalty will be based on performance in calendar year 2013, so providers should plan for decreased reimbursement from the CMS in 2015 if they do not report these data in 2013. In addition to a change from incentives to participate to penalties for not participating, it is likely that PQRS will move from a model of reimbursement adjustments based on reporting to one based on actual performance.

MECHANISMS BY WHICH PMs MIGHT AFFECT QUALITY

In addition to merely rewarding high-quality care, VBP has the potential to affect quality of care, whether assessed as a function of how often recommended processes of care are adhered to or as a function of how often desired outcomes are achieved. Physicians can be induced by financial incentives to alter their clinical

Table 1
Selected NQF-endorsed performance measures related to critical care

Title (NQF Measure Number)	Description	Risk-adjusted	Type of Measure
Empiric antibiotic for community-acquired bacterial pneumonia (NQF 96)	Percentage of patients aged 18 y and older with a diagnosis of community-acquired bacterial pneumonia with an appropriate empiric antibiotic prescribed	No	Process
Ventilator-associated pneumonia for ICU and high-risk nursery patients (NQF 140)	Ventilator-associated pneumonias in ICU and high-risk nursery patients per 1000 ventilator days	Yes	Outcome
Initial antibiotic selection for community-acquired pneumonia in immunocompetent adults (NQF 147)	Percentage of pneumonia patients 18 y of age or older selected for initial receipts of antibiotics for community-acquired pneumonia	No	Process
Blood cultures performed in the emergency department before initial antibiotic received in hospital (NQF 148)	Percentage of pneumonia patients 18 y of age and older who have had blood cultures performed in the emergency department before initial antibiotic received in hospital	No	Process
Initial antibiotic received within 6 h of hospital arrival (NQF 151)	Percentage of pneumonia patients 18 y of age and older who receive their first dose of antibiotics within 6 h after arrival at the hospital	No	Process
Proportion admitted to the ICU in the last 30 d of life (NQF 213)	Percentage of patients who died from cancer admitted to the ICU in the last 30 d of life	No	Process
Proportion not admitted to hospice (NQF 215)	Percentage of patients who died from cancer not admitted to hospice	No	Process
Vital signs for community-acquired pneumonia (NQF 232)	Percentage of patients aged 18 y and older with a diagnosis of community-acquired bacterial pneumonia with vital signs (temperature, pulse, respiratory rate, and blood pressure) documented and reviewed	No	Process
Assessment of oxygen saturation for community-acquired bacterial pneumonia (NQF 233)	Percentage of patients aged 18 y and older with the diagnosis of community-acquired bacterial pneumonia with oxygen saturation documented and reviewed	No	Process

Bacterial pneumonia (NQF 279)	This measure is used to assess the number of admissions for bacterial pneumonia per 100,000 population	Yes	Outcome
Ventilator bundle (NQF 302)	Percentage of ICU patients on mechanical ventilation at time of survey for whom all 4 elements of the ventilator bundle are documented: • Head of bed elevation 30° or greater • Daily "sedation interruption" and daily assessment of readiness to extubate • Stress ulcer disease (peptic ulcer disease) prophylaxis • Deep vein thrombosis prophylaxis	No	Composite process measure
Severity-standardized average length of stay–special care (NQF 332)	Standardized average length of stay for special inpatient care (ie, care provided in ICUs)	Yes	Outcome
Pediatric ICU (PICU) severity adjusted length of stay (NQF 334)	The number of days between PICU admission and PICU discharge	Yes	Outcome
PICU unplanned readmission rate (NQF 335)	The total number of patients requiring unscheduled readmission to the ICU within 24 h of discharge or transfer	No	Outcome
PICU pain assessment on admission (NQF 341)	Percentage of PICU patients receiving pain assessment on admission	No	Process
PICU periodic pain assessment (NQF 342)	Percentage of PICU patients receiving periodic pain assessment	No	Process
PICU standardized mortality ratio (NQF 343)	Ratio of actual deaths over predicted deaths for PICU patients	Yes	Outcome
Death among surgical inpatients with serous, treatable complications (NQF 351)	Percentage of cases having developed specified complications of care with an in-hospital death	Yes	Outcome
Blood cultures performed in pneumonia (NQF 356)	Percent of pneumonia patients, age 18 y or older, transferred or admitted to the ICU within 24 h of hospital arrival who had blood cultures performed within 24 h before or 24 h after arrival at the hospital	No	Process

(*continued on next page*)

Table 1
(continued)

Title (NQF Measure Number)	Description	Risk-adjusted	Type of Measure
Hospital 30-d standardized mortality rate after pneumonia hospitalization (NQF 468)	The measure estimates a hospital-level risk-standardized mortality rate defined as death for any cause within 30 d of the admission date for the index hospitalization for patients discharged from the hospital with a principal diagnosis of pneumonia	Yes	Outcome
Severe sepsis and septic shock: management bundle (NQF 500)	Number of patients who meet criteria for severe sepsis and septic who had orders for 1. Blood, urine, and appropriate cultures 2. Broad-spectrum antibiotic(s) 3. Fluids and 4. Measurement of lactate clearance	No	Composite process measure
Confirmation of endotracheal tube placement (NQF 501)	Any time an endotracheal tube is placed into an airway before arrival or in the emergency department there should be some method attempted to confirm endotracheal tube placement	No	Process
Anticoagulation for acute pulmonary embolism (NQF 503)	Anticoagulation ordered for acute pulmonary embolism patients	No	Process
30-d All-cause risk standardized readmission rate after pneumonia hospitalization (NQF 506)	Hospital-specific 30-d all-cause risk standardized readmission rate following hospitalization for pneumonia among Medicare beneficiaries aged 65 y or older at the time of index hospitalization	Yes	Outcome
Ultrasound guidance for internal jugular central venous catheter placement (NQF 666)	Percent of adult patients aged 18 y and older with an internal jugular central venous catheter placed in the emergency department under ultrasound guidance	No	Process
ICU length of stay (NQF 702)	For all patients admitted to the ICU, total duration of time spent in the ICU until time of discharge; both observed and risk-adjusted length of stay reported	Yes	Outcome

	with the predicted length of stay measured using the Intensive Care Outcomes Model–Length-of-Stay		
Intensive care: in-hospital mortality rate (NQF 703)	For all adult patients admitted to the ICU, the percentage of patients whose hospital outcome is death; both observed and risk-adjusted mortality rates are reported with predicted rates based on the Intensive Care Outcomes Model–Mortality	Yes	Outcome
Proportion of patients hospitalized with stroke that have a potentially avoidable complication (NQF 705)	Percent of adult population aged 18–65 y who were admitted to a hospital with stroke, were followed for 1 month after discharge, and had 1 or more potentially avoidable complications	Yes	Outcome
Proportion of patients hospitalized with pneumonia that have a potentially avoidable complication (NQF 708)	Percent of adult population aged 18–65 y who were admitted to a hospital with pneumonia, were followed for 1 month after discharge, and had 1 or more potentially avoidable complications	Yes	Outcome
Patients admitted to ICU who have care preferences documented (NQF 1626)	Percentage of vulnerable adults admitted to ICU who survive at least 48 h who have their care preferences documented within 48 h or documentation as to why this was not done	No	Process
Hospice and palliative care—treatment preferences (NQF 1641)	Percentage of patients with chart documentation of preferences for life-sustaining treatments	No	Process
Hospital-wide all-cause unplanned readmission rate (NQF 1789)	This measure estimates the hospital-level, risk-standardized rate of unplanned, all-cause readmission after admission for any eligible condition within 30 d of hospital discharge for patients aged 18 and older	Yes	Outcome

Data from National Quality Forum. NQF Endorses Pulmonary and Critical Care Measures. National Quality Forum, Washington DC; 2011. Available at: http://www.qualityforum.org/News_And_Resources/Press_Releases/2012/NQF_Endorses_Pulmonary_and_Critical_Care_Measures.aspx.

Table 2
Measures included in inpatient prospective payment system for value-based purchasing program

Fiscal Year	2013	2014	2015
Process measures—relative weight in VBP	70%	45%	20%
Acute myocardial infarction			
AMI-7a: fibrinolytic therapy within 30 min of hospital arrival	X	X	X
AMI-8: primary PCI within 90 min of hospital arrival	X	X	X
AMI-10: statin prescribed at discharge			X
Congestive heart failure			
HF-1: discharge instructions	X	X	X
Pneumonia			
PN-3b: blood cultures performed in an emergency department before initial antibiotics for ICU patients	X	X	X
PN-6: initial antibiotic selection for CAP	X	X	X
Surgical care			
SCIP-Inf-1: prophylactic antibiotics within 1 h before incision	X	X	X
SCIP-Inf-2: prophylactic antibiotic choice	X	X	X
SCIP-Inf-3: prophylactic antibiotics discontinued within 24 h	X	X	X
SCIP-Inf-4: cardiac surgery patients with controlled 6 AM postoperative glucose	X	X	X
SCIP-Inf-9: urinary catheter removed on postoperative day 1 or 2		X	X
SCIP-Card-2: surgery patients continued on β-blockers postoperatively	X	X	X
SCIP-VTE-1: surgery patients with VTE prophylaxis ordered	X	X	
SCIP-VTE-2: surgery patients receiving VTE prophylaxis within 24 h	X	X	X
Patient experience measures—relative weight in VBP	30%	30%	30%
Hospital Consumer Assessment of Healthcare Providers and Systems	X	X	X
Outcome measures—relative weight in VBP	—	25%	30%
AMI—30-d mortality rate		X	X
Heart failure—30-d mortality rate		X	X
Pneumonia—30-d mortality rate		X	X
CLABSI			X
AHRQ PSI-90: complication/patient safety index			X
Efficiency measures—relative weight in VBP	—	—	20%
Medicare spending per beneficiary			X

Abbreviations: AHRQ, Agency for Healthcare Research and Quality; AMI, acute myocardial infarction; CAP, community-acquired pneumonia; CLABSI, ventral line-associated bloodstream infection; ICU, intensive care unit; PCI, percutaneous coronary intervention; VTE, venous thromboembolism.

The PSI-90 includes pressure ulcer, iatrogenic pneumothorax, CVC-related bloodstream infection, postoperative hip fracture, postoperative hemorrhage/hematoma, postoperative physiologic and metabolic derangements, postoperative respiratory failure, postoperative pulmonary embolism and/or deep venous thrombosis, postoperative sepsis, postoperative wound dehiscence, and accidental puncture or laceration. X means this is part of VBP in that year and Blank means it is not.

practices. Thus, VBP may directly improve quality of care by incentivizing clinicians to use recommended processes care or by inducing them to institute locally developed processes for improving relevant outcomes. Similarly, VBP may incentivize structural changes that are believed to lead to better outcomes. For example, the

Box 2
Hospital-acquired conditions in the CMS inpatient prospective payer system

- Foreign object retained after surgery
- Air embolism
- Blood incompatibility
- Pressure ulcers
  - Stage III
  - Stage IV
- Falls and trauma
  - Fracture
  - Dislocation
  - Intracranial injury
  - Crushing injury
  - Burn
  - Other injuries
- Catheter-associated urinary tract infection
- Vascular catheter–associated infection
- Manifestations of poor glycemic control
  - Diabetic ketoacidosis
  - Nonketotic hyperosmolar coma
  - Hypoglycemic coma
  - Secondary diabetes with ketoacidosis
  - Secondary diabetes with hyperosmolarity
- Surgical site infection
  - After coronary artery bypass graft
    - Mediastinitis
  - After certain orthopedic procedures
    - Spine
    - Neck
    - Shoulder
    - Elbow
  - After bariatric surgery for obesity
  - After cardiac implantable electronic devices procedures
- Iatrogenic pneumothorax associated with vascular catheters
- Deep vein thrombosis/pulmonary embolism following certain orthopedic procedures
  - Total knee replacement
  - Hip replacement

Data from Department of Health and Human Resources. Centers for Medicare and Medicaid Services. Hospital-Acquired Conditions (HAC) in Acute Inpatient Prospective Payment System (IPPS) Hospitals. Available at: http://www.cms.gov/Medicare/Medicare-Fee-for-Service-Payment/HospitalAcqCond/downloads/hacfactsheet.pdf.

Table 3
Selected PQRS measures related to critical care

Title (Measure Number)	Description
Coronary artery disease: antiplatelet therapy (6)	Percentage of patients aged 18 y and older with a diagnosis of coronary artery disease seen within a 12-mo period who were prescribed aspirin or clopidogrel
Perioperative care: timing of antibiotic prophylaxis—ordering physician (20)	Percentage of surgical patients aged 18 y and older undergoing procedures with the indications for prophylactic parenteral antibiotics, who have an order for prophylactic parenteral antibiotic to be given within 1 h (if fluoroquinolone or vancomycin, 2 h), before the surgical incision (or start of procedure when no incision is required)
Perioperative care: selection of prophylactic antibiotic—first- or second-generation cephalosporin (21)	Percentage of surgical patients aged 18 y and older undergoing procedures with the indications for a first OR second-generation cephalosporin prophylactic antibiotic who had an order for cefazolin OR cefuroxime for antimicrobial prophylaxis
Perioperative care: discontinuation of prophylactic antibiotics (noncardiac procedures) (22)	Percentage of noncardiac surgical patients aged 18 y and older undergoing procedures with the indications for prophylactic parenteral antibiotics AND who received a prophylactic parenteral antibiotic, who have an order for discontinuation of prophylactic parenteral antibiotics within 24 h of surgical end time
Perioperative care: venous thromboembolism prophylaxis (when indicated in ALL patients) (23)	Percentage of patients aged 18 y and older undergoing procedures for which venous thromboembolism prophylaxis is indicated in all patients, who had an order for low-molecular-weight heparin, low-dose unfractionated heparin, adjusted-dose warfarin, fondaparinux, or mechanical prophylaxis to be given within 24 h before incision time or within 24 h after surgery end time
Aspirin at arrival for acute myocardial infarction (28)	Percentage of patients with an emergency department discharge diagnosis of acute myocardial infarction who had documentation of receiving aspirin
Perioperative care: timely administration of prophylactic parenteral antibioitcs (30)	Percentage of surgical patients aged 18 y and older who receive an anesthetic when undergoing procedures with the indications for prophylactic parenteral antibiotics for whom administration of prophylactic parenteral antibiotic ordered fluoroquinolone or vancomycin, 2 h) before the surgical incision (or start of procedure when no incision is required)

(*continued on next page*)

Table 3
(continued)

Title (Measure Number)	Description
Stroke and stroke rehabilitation: deep vein thrombosis prophylaxis for ischemic stroke or intracranial hemorrhage (31)	Percentage of patients aged 18 y and older with a diagnosis of ischemic stroke or intracranial hemorrhage who were administered deep vein thrombosis prophylaxis by end of hospital day 2
Stroke and stroke rehabilitation: discharged on antithrombotic therapy (32)	Percentage of patients aged 18 y and older with a diagnosis of ischemic stroke or transient ischemic attack who were prescribed antithrombotic therapy at discharge
Stroke and stroke rehabilitation: screening for dysphagia (35)	Percentage of patients aged 18 y and older with a diagnosis of ischemic stroke or intracranial hemorrhage who receive any foods, fluids, or medication by mouth for whom a dysphagia screening was performed before by oral intake in accordance with a dysphagia screening tool approved by the institution in which the patient is receiving care
Stroke and stroke rehabilitation: rehabilitation services ordered (36)	Percentage of patients aged 18 y and older with a diagnosis of ischemic stroke or intracranial hemorrhage for whom occupational, physical or speech rehabilitation services were ordered at or before inpatient discharge, OR documentation that no rehabilitation services are indicated at or before inpatient discharge
Coronary artery bypass graft: preoperative β-blocker in patients with isolated coronary artery bypass graft surgery (44)	Percentage of patients aged 18 y and older undergoing isolated coronary artery bypass graft surgery who received a β-blocker within 24 h before surgical incision
Perioperative care: discontinuation of prophylactic antibiotics (cardiac procedures) (45)	Percentage of cardiac surgical patients aged 18 y and older undergoing procedures with the indications for prophylactic antibiotics AND who received a prophylactic antibiotic, who have an order for discontinuation of prophylactic antibiotics within 48 h of surgical end time
Emergency medicine: 12-lead ECG performed for nontraumatic chest pain (54)	Percentage of patients aged 40 y and older with an emergency department discharge diagnosis of nontraumatic chest pain who had a 12-lead ECG performed
Emergency medicine: 12-lead ECG performed for syncope (55)	Percentage of patients aged 60 y and older with an emergency department discharge diagnosis of syncope who had a 12-lead ECG performed
Emergency medicine: CAP: vital signs (56)	Percentage of patients aged 18 y and older with a diagnosis of community-acquired bacterial pneumonia with vital signs documented and reviewed

(continued on next page)

Table 3
(continued)

Title (Measure Number)	Description
Emergency medicine: CAP: assessment of oxygen saturation (57)	Percentage of patients aged 18 y and older with a diagnosis of community-acquired bacterial pneumonia with oxygen saturation documented and reviewed
Emergency medicine: CAP: assessment of mental status (58)	Percentage of patients aged 18 y and older with a diagnosis of community-acquired bacterial pneumonia with mental status assessed
Emergency medicine: CAP: empiric antibiotic (59)	Percentage of patients aged 18 y and older with a diagnosis of community-acquired bacterial pneumonia with an appropriate empiric antibiotic prescribed
Prevention of catheter-related bloodstream infections: CVC insertion protocol (76)	Percentage of patients, regardless of age, who undergo CVC insertion for whom CVC was inserted with all elements of maximal sterile barrier technique (cap AND mask AND sterile gown AND sterile gloves AND a large sterile sheet AND hand hygiene AND 2% chlorhexidine for cutaneous antisepsis [or acceptable alternative antiseptics per current guideline]) followed
Perioperative temperature management (193)	Percentage of patients, regardless of age, undergoing surgical or therapeutic procedures under general or neuraxial anesthesia of 60 min duration or longer, except patients undergoing cardiopulmonary bypass, for whom either active warming was used intraoperatively for the purpose of maintaining normothermia, OR at least 1 body temperature equal to or greater than 36°C (or 96.8°F) was recorded within the 30 min immediately before or the 15 min immediately after anesthesia end time
Anticoagulation for acute pulmonary embolus patients (252)	Anticoagulation ordered for patients who have been discharged from the emergency department with a diagnosis of acute pulmonary embolus

Abbreviations: CAP, community-acquired pneumonia; CVC, central venous catheter.

Data from Department of Health and Human Resources. Centers for Medicare and Medicaid Services. 2012 Physician Quality Reporting System and Electronic Prescribing (eRx) Incentive Program Group Practice Reporting Option (GPRO): Participation for the Incentive Payment Made Simple. Available at: http://www.cms.gov/Outreach-and-Education/Medicare-Learning-Network-MLN/MLNProducts/Downloads/2012GPROMadeSimple.pdf.

CMS meaningful use program has provided financial rewards to medical practices and hospitals for implementation of EHRs. Although not relevant to VBP programs that have an impact on essentially all providers (eg, CMS programs), VBP programs that target selected hospitals or medical practices could theoretically induce competitors of the targeted entities to improve their quality to ensure that they remain competitive.

More than one expert has written about the potential unintended negative consequences that could result from VBP programs.[29,30] There are several mechanisms by which VBP could reduce the quality of care. The first is by incentivizing processes of care that are recommended but for which the recommendation is erroneous. For example, after a few positive studies were published, tight insulin control for critically ill patients was widely recommended and became accepted as a quality measure by the Surviving Sepsis Campaign and the CMS Surgical Care Improvement Program. Later research demonstrated that tight glucose in critically ill patients resulted in increased patient mortality.[31] Had there been large incentives associated with these campaigns, there would have been higher adherence and, as a result, greater patient harm. This is by no means a unique occurrence, because other strongly recommended processes of care, such as routine performance of blood cultures on patients admitted to the hospital with pneumonia and perioperative β-blockade, have also fallen by the wayside as knowledge has advanced. Another potential risk of financially incentivizing care is that truly beneficial processes of care will be provided to a subset of patients in whom there is a greater risk of harm or, at the least, limited chance of benefit. If nothing else, such practices waste resources. It is common to see patients with terminal illness in whom a cardiologist or primary care physician dutifully continues the expensive and useless medications for lipid and blood pressure control. This would likely increase if meaningful incentives were in place.

There is also concern providing a disproportionate reward for certain processes of care might result in excessive attention to that process and inadequate attention to other important aspects of care, the health care equivalent of "teaching to the test." Although there is limited evidence this issue has led to diminished quality of care, the potential for this phenomenon exists. For example, it has been estimated that a critical care nurse would have to spend approximately 2 hours of a 12-hour shift purely on work related to tight insulin control of 2 patients.[32] What important work might go undone in such a situation?

One of the most credible concerns is that VBP could result in worsened care by increasing the frequency of cherry picking. There are patient populations in whom it is more difficult to achieve high rates of adherence to recommended processes of care (socioeconomically disadvantaged patients) and populations in whom it is more difficult to achieve optimum outcomes (patients with multiple comorbidities and more complex involvement of even a single disease). Avoidance of such patients has been demonstrated after the institution of public reporting of cardiac surgery outcomes in New York, despite there being no direct financial implications associated with the reports.[33] It is likely that introducing meaningful financial incentives for either processes or outcomes would exacerbate this phenomenon, limiting the availability of needed care for any patients who might diminish a hospital or provider's ability to hit their numbers. Similarly, tertiary-care hospitals that care for some of the most difficult and complex patients could be harmed by a VBP plan that relies on poorly conceived measures, for example, outcomes measures that do not incorporate sound risk adjustment methodology.

VBP can also result in worsened care indirectly. There is often a correlation between hospitals' financial status and their quality. Hospitals that are profitable have more dollars available to invest in technology and staff to maintain and improve quality. Alternatively, many of the hospitals with lower measured quality are financially underperforming, often serving a lower socioeconomic demographic, and, therefore, possessing a poor payer mix.[34] If these hospitals see their reimbursement drop even further as a result of financial penalties, their quality might decline as they become more financially unstable.

Perhaps the most insidious potential negative consequence of VBP is its necessary reliance on financial incentives and penalties that could contribute to erosion of the altruism and beneficence that should be at the foundation of medical practice.[30] Given the number of other threats to these core values, such as declining reimbursement, the loss of autonomy, and the promulgation of work hour limits, such an effect would be difficult to measure but are still a concern.

EVIDENCE OF EFFECT OF VBP ON QUALITY IN GENERAL

Despite the enthusiasm with which public and private payers have embraced VBP, there is surprisingly little convincing evidence that VBP can predictably result in robust improvements in quality of care. In 2003, one of California's largest health plans began paying physicians bonuses for performance related to 10 quality metrics.[35] Although improvements were seen in the rates of 3 screening processes of care, the improvements were modest (2%–5%) and were only better than a control group of physicians for 2 of the metrics. Lindenauer and colleagues[36] evaluated the changes in performance related to 10 publicly reported hospital process measures over 2 years and compared the results among 207 hospitals that were participating in a CMS pay-for-performance demonstration project with a control group of 406 hospitals that were not participating. After adjustment for hospital characteristics and baseline performance, both groups of hospitals demonstrated steady improvement during the study period, with the pay-for-performance hospitals showing a 2.6% to 4.1% greater improvement. Hospitals with the lowest performance at baseline had the greatest improvement. A subsequent report examining the changes in 30-day mortality associated with the same CMS demonstration project, however, found no improvements among the pay-for-performance hospitals compared with nonparticipating control hospitals.[37] A review of hospital pay-for-performance programs concluded that most published studies had methodologic flaws, such as lack of a control group of hospitals, but modest improvements in quality as assessed by process measures are often seen.[38] In summary, although there has been variability in the success of various pay-for-performance programs, modest improvements in quality (defined by adherence to recommended processes of care) are often achieved. There is, however, essentially no evidence that pay-for-performance programs results in improvements in patient outcomes.[39] Factors that likely contribute to the success of any pay-for-performance program include the magnitude of the potential incentive relative to the cost of implementing quality improvement efforts, the baseline performance of the hospital, and the financial ability of the hospital or provider to invest in efforts to improve quality.

EVIDENCE OF EFFECT OF VBP ON QUALITY IN CRITICAL CARE

As with the effects of VBP on quality in general, there are few studies that evaluate the influence on care for critically ill patients. As discussed are addressed in both the article by Watson and Scales as well as the article by Tropello and colleagues in this issue, there are many examples of quality improvement projects organized around consortiums (eg, Keystone [http://mhakeystonecenter.org/]), grants (eg, Surviving Sepsis Campaign), and within health systems or individual hospitals. It is less clear, however, that specific VBP programs are influential drivers of these programs or downstream outcomes.

Data on the effects of the actual CMS VBP program are unavailable because reimbursement based on performance is not in effect until FY 2013. The effect of reporting alone, however, may allow for inferences about the possible influence on quality of care. The AHRQ annually prepares the National Healthcare Quality Report[40] as required by Congress. This reports on trends in the quality of health care and considers trends significant if there is an average annual trend of change of at least 1% per year with an inferential test for trend significance (*P*<.1). The 2011 report[40] includes data from 2002 to 2008—a period when reporting from hospitals was required but before implementation of reimbursement based on performance. Significant improvements were noted in process measures for quality of care for acute myocardial infarction, including timeliness of cardiac reperfusion, and the overall impatient mortality rate decreased significantly. Recommended care for pneumonia also improved, with 93% of hospital patients receiving all 5 processes of care (timing of antibiotics, choice of antibiotics, blood cultures, and influenza and pneumococcal vaccinations). There was also a significant decrease in the inpatient mortality rate for pneumonia over this time. Pressure ulcer rates fell among nursing home residents but actually increased among hospitalized patients. Within the Surgical Care Improvement Project (SCIP) measures, timing of prophylactic antibiotics significantly improved and by 2009 86% of surgery patients received all appropriate care. Rates of postoperative pulmonary embolism and/or deep venous thrombosis worsened, however, and there was no change in the rate of postoperative respiratory failure. Across all measures of quality in the report, almost 60% showed improvement but the median change was only 2.5% per year.

One of the earliest moves toward payers attempting to influence the quality of provided care was promoted by the Leapfrog Group. Formed in 2000, this group of large employers began discussing how they could collaborate to influence health care quality and cost.[41] One of the initial foci of the Leapfrog Group was the recommendation for full-time intensivist staffing in ICUs—also known as the ICU physician staffing standard (IPS). This recommendation was based on several studies suggesting improved adherence to evidence-based medicine and improved outcomes when such a model was used. Implementation of this model has been incomplete due to several barriers, including the associated start-up costs and institutional politics of beginning such a program. A recent before-and-after analysis of implementation of the IPS at a 308-bed community teaching hospital supports the value of this staffing model as a structural PM.[42] At baseline, any physician could admit and manage a patient in the hospital's 15-bed ICU with required consultation for mechanically ventilated patients and discretionary consults for all other patients. After IPS implementation, board-certified intensivists assumed administrative and medical management responsibilities in the ICU. All medical patients were admitted to the intensivists' service and all surgical patients in the ICU for more than 24 hours required consultation. Multidisciplinary rounds were also incorporated with IPS. On-site nocturnal ICU coverage was provided by house staff. After implementation of the IPS, there was a significant decrease in the number of CLABSIs (8.5 per 1000 to 1.60 per 1000 catheter days, *P*<.0002), the number of ventilator days per patient (7.9–3.4, *P* value not reported), the rate of ventilator associated pneumonia (1.03 per 100 ventilator days to 0.38, *P*<.0002), and ICU length of stay (3.5–2.7 days, *P*<.002). There was no significant effect on ward or hospital length of stay and there was a nonsignificant increase in mortality noted (7.0%–8.4%). The investigators estimated that the IPS resulted in avoided costs during hospitalization of $1,777,052 in 1 year and a return on investment (based on ICU physician salaries) of 105%. These findings seem to corroborate the results of a hypothetical model of the financial effects of implementation of the IPS model.[43] Despite these findings, such a staffing model is not incorporated into the CMS VBP program and, based on a 2007 survey, only 30% of hospitals met the IPS standards.[44]

One area of particular interest for surgical disciplines has been the elimination of wrong-site procedures. In 2002, the American College of Surgeons recommended the development of institutional guidelines that ensure correct patient, correct site, and correct procedure.[45] Beginning July 1, 2004, The Joint Commission required a Universal Protocol, including preprocedure verification, surgical site marking, and a preprocedure time out.[46] A study of self-reported wrong-site and wrong-patient procedures sought to determine if there was an association between such events and the requirement for the Universal Protocol.[47] Although events were self-reported, the database was from a professional liability company that provided incentives for timely reporting of adverse events and complications by covered physicians. Neither the number of wrong-patient or wrong-site reports was changed after The Joint Commission requirement. The peak number of wrong-patient cases occurred in 2004 and 2005 and the peak for wrong-site procedures occurred in 2005 and 2007. Although this could represent a greater willingness to report such events in the Universal Protocol period, the total number of occurrences reported and the total number of resulting claims or lawsuits were not changed, suggesting consistency of reporting. Regardless, these data did not provide evidence of a decrease in wrong-patient or wrong-site procedures as a result of enactment of this regulation.

As discussed previously, CLABSIs have been considered an HAC since 2005, with no reimbursement for provision of care since October 2008. The Centers for Disease Control estimated the change in CLABSI rates from 2001 to 2009 based on sampled data from the National Nosocomial Infection Surveillance System.[48] In 2001, it was estimated that there were 3.64 CLABSIs per 1000 line days in ICUs—resulting in 43,000 CLABSIs. In 2009, the central line use rate was similar to that observed in 2001, but the rate of CLABSIs dropped to 1.65 infections per 1000 line days or an estimated 18,000 CLABSIs. This is an estimated 58% reduction in the number of CLABSIs in 2009 compared with in 2001. The investigators estimated that these avoided infections represented 3000 to 6000 lives and $414 million in health care costs saved in 2009 alone. It is unclear the specific effects changes in HAC reporting and reimbursement had on CLABSI rates.

THE FUTURE OF VBP IN CRITICAL CARE

There are few data to support or not support the use of VBP to improve quality in ICUs. The documented cost associated with critical care, the variations in processes and outcomes of care, and the evidence that quality-improvement programs have been successful in improving health care value make it likely, however, that VBP will address ICU care in the near future. There are several NQF-endorsed measures that may be ready targets for inclusion in VBP. Some, such as adherence to the Leapfrog IPS, would require significant up-front investment by hospitals, which may create reluctance on the part of influential groups, such as the American Hospital Association, to endorse its enactment. Additionally, the demand for critical care physicians already exceeds supply and this gap is likely to widen.[4]

It is unlikely that high-level evidence showing the benefit of VBP targeting critical care will be developed before its inclusion into the CMS program. As a result, there will have to be input and guidance from providers and their specialty societies as to the targets most likely to improve health care quality and the unintended consequences that could arise. For example, the initial DRG-penalty related to excess readmissions seems to affect hospitals treating poorer patients more than hospitals treating fewer such patients.[49] Hospitals with the greatest number of poor patients were more likely to receive any penalty and were twice as likely to receive the maximum penalty compared with hospitals treating the fewest poor patients (12% of hospitals vs 6% of hospitals). Prior studies have found that patient socioeconomic status is independently associated with the risk of readmission.[50,51] The primary drivers of variability in readmission rates seem to be the characteristics of a hospital's patient population and the resources of the community in which it is located, rather than the quality of care provided.[51] Furthermore, a recent systematic review reported that, on average, only 27% of readmissions were preventable.[52] Additionally, although total readmission rates vary among hospitals, there are data suggesting that preventable readmission rates are consistent across hospitals.[53] It remains to be seen if this program will cause the penalized hospitals to re-engineer their delivery of care and improve outcomes or if the hospitals with the worst payer mix will suffer from even lower revenue resulting in less ability to improve care.

Two paired NQF-endorsed measures that are possible candidates for implementation in VBP are worthy of comment: Intensive care: In-hospital mortality rate and Intensive Care Unit Length-of-Stay. These risk-adjusted measures are intended to address variation in outcome and resource use among ICUs in an effort to improve quality. Although laudable in the motivation, there are concerns for deleterious unintended consequences. First, the in-hospital mortality rate is tied to hospital discharge—a landmark that may be prone to discharge bias—rather than measuring mortality at some fixed point, such as 30 days or 90 days after admission. It is also unclear that shortening ICU length of stay reduces costs significantly because the difference in cost for the final ICU day and the first day outside the ICU in the hospital is marginal.[54] Focus on this measure, however, could result in premature ICU discharge and, ultimately, prolonged hospitalization. Additionally, the emphasis on mortality could reduce the likelihood of honest discussion about goals of care and create a barrier to consideration of palliative interventions. This shift could increase costs associated with care at the end of life and move further from the goal of patient centeredness. Finally, a recent study of 137 hospitals directly challenges the proposition that these measures, as currently specified, adequately address value.[55] This study observed variation in observed to expected ratios for hospital mortality (mean 0.90 [95% prediction interval, 0.50 to 1.30]) and length of stay (mean 1.12 [95% prediction interval, 0.60 to 1.64]). Similarly, there was observed variation among hospitals in rate of discharges to long-term acute care hospitals (LTACHs) (range 0%–50%). Most relevant to these measures, 14% of the variation in hospital mortality index and 37% of the variation in length of stay index was explained by the LTACH transfer rate. Considering that annual costs of care for LTACH patients increased from $484 million in 1997 to $1.325 billion in 2006 and that mortality after LTACH admission remains high (52% at 1 year in 2004–2006),[56] measures that might promote such transfers may not improve overall health care value.

SUMMARY

Regardless of changes in leadership in the federal government, it is likely that VBP will expand within the CMS inpatient payer system. Currently, VBP in critical care focuses on health care acquired conditions and cardiovascular disease. Despite a lack of high-level evidence supporting its beneficial effect on outcomes for patients, including those with critical illness, it is likely that the scope of VBP will expand, with its effect measured after its implementation. Considering the central role of NQF in endorsing PMs for inclusion in the CMS VBP program, attention to proposed and endorsed measures may foreshadow the future of VBP in ICUs.

REFERENCES

1. Martin AB, Lassman D, Washington B, et al. Growth in US health spending remained slow in 2010; health share of gross domestic product was unchanged from 2009. Health Aff (Millwood) 2012;31(1):208–19.

2. Halpern NA, Pastores SM. Critical care medicine in the United States 2000-2005: an analysis of bed numbers, occupancy rates, payer mix, and costs. Crit Care Med 2010;38(1):65–71.
3. Noseworthy TW, Konopad E, Shustack A, et al. Cost accounting of adult intensive care: methods and human and capital inputs. Crit Care Med 1996;24(7):1168–72.
4. Angus DC, Kelley MA, Schmitz RJ, et al. Caring for the critically ill patient. Current and projected workforce requirements for care of the critically ill and patients with pulmonary disease: can we meet the requirements of an aging population? JAMA 2000;284(21):2762–70.
5. Lubitz JD, Riley GF. Trends in Medicare payments in the last year of life. N Engl J Med 1993;328(15):1092–6.
6. Barnato AE, McClellan MB, Kagay CR, et al. Trends in inpatient treatment intensity among Medicare beneficiaries at the end of life. Health Serv Res 2004;39(2): 363–75.
7. Donchin Y, Gopher D, Olin M, et al. A look into the nature and causes of human errors in the intensive care unit. 1995. Qual Saf Health Care 2003;12(2):143–7.
8. Ventilation with lower tidal volumes as compared with traditional tidal volumes for acute lung injury and the acute respiratory distress syndrome. The Acute Respiratory Distress Syndrome Network. N Engl J Med 2000;342(18):1301–8.
9. Kumar A, Roberts D, Wood KE, et al. Duration of hypotension before initiation of effective antimicrobial therapy is the critical determinant of survival in human septic shock. Crit Care Med 2006;34(6):1589–96.
10. Pronovost P, Needham D, Berenholtz S, et al. An intervention to decrease catheter-related bloodstream infections in the ICU. N Engl J Med 2006;355(26): 2725–32.
11. Berenholtz SM, Pham JC, Thompson DA, et al. Collaborative cohort study of an intervention to reduce ventilator-associated pneumonia in the intensive care unit. Infect Control Hosp Epidemiol 2011;32(4):305–14.
12. Girard TD, Kress JP, Fuchs BD, et al. Efficacy and safety of a paired sedation and ventilator weaning protocol for mechanically ventilated patients in intensive care (Awakening and Breathing Controlled trial): a randomised controlled trial. Lancet 2008;371(9607):126–34.
13. Needham DM, Colantuoni E, Mendez-Tellez PA, et al. Lung protective mechanical ventilation and two year survival in patients with acute lung injury: prospective cohort study. BMJ 2012;344:e2124.
14. Mikkelsen ME, Dedhiya PM, Kalhan R, et al. Potential reasons why physicians underuse lung-protective ventilation: a retrospective cohort study using physician documentation. Respir Care 2008;53(4):455–61.
15. Rubenfeld GD, Cooper C, Carter G, et al. Barriers to providing lung-protective ventilation to patients with acute lung injury. Crit Care Med 2004;32(6):1289–93.
16. Porter ME. What is value in health care? N Engl J Med 2010;363(26):2477–81.
17. Eldridge GN, Korda H. Value-based purchasing: the evidence. Am J Manag Care 2011;17(8):e310–3.
18. 2010 National P4P survey: executive summary. Med-Vantage, Inc; 2012. Available at: http://www.imshealth.com/ims/Global/Content/Solutions/Healthcare%20Analytics%20and%20Services/Payer%20Solutions/Survey_Exec_Sum.pdf.
19. President's Advisory Commission on Consumer Protection and Quality in the Health Care Industry. 1998. Available at: http://archive.ahrq.gov/hcqual/final/append_a.html.
20. Proposed revisions to payment policies under the physician fee schedule, and other Part B payment policies for CY 2008. Fed Regist 2007;72(133):38196–9.

21. NQF: governance and leadership. 2012. Available at: http://www.qualityforum.org/About_NQF/Governance_and_Leadership.aspx. Accessed September 7, 2012.
22. NQF: consensus development process. 2012. Available at: http://www.qualityforum.org/Measuring_Performance/Consensus_Development_Process.aspx. Accessed September 7, 2012.
23. NQF: measure evaluation criteria. 2012. Available at: http://www.qualityforum.org/Measuring_Performance/Submitting_Standards/Measure_Evaluation_Criteria.aspx. Accessed September 7, 2012.
24. NQF-endorsed standards. 2012. Available at: http://www.qualityforum.org/Measures_List.aspx. Accessed September 7, 2012.
25. Hospital value-based purchasing. 2012. Available at: http://www.qualityforum.org/Measures_List.aspx. Accessed September 7, 2012.
26. Readmissions reduction program. 2012. Available at: http://cms.gov/Medicare/Medicare-Fee-for-Service-Payment/AcuteInpatientPPS/Readmissions-Reduction-Program.html/. Accessed September 7, 2012.
27. Hospital-acquired conditions. 2012. Available at: http://www.cms.gov/Medicare/Medicare-Fee-for-Service-Payment/HospitalAcqCond/index.html?redirect=/HospitalAcqCond/. Accessed September 7, 2012.
28. Physician quality reporting system. 2012. Available at: http://www.cms.gov/Medicare/Quality-Initiatives-Patient-Assessment-Instruments/PQRS/index.html?redirect=/pqrs. Accessed September 7, 2012.
29. Epstein AM, Lee TH, Hamel MB. Paying physicians for high-quality care. N Engl J Med 2004;350(4):406–10.
30. Fisher ES. Paying for performance—risks and recommendations. N Engl J Med 2006;355(18):1845–7.
31. Finfer S, Chittock DR, Su SY, et al. Intensive versus conventional glucose control in critically ill patients. N Engl J Med 2009;360(13):1283–97.
32. Wachter R. ICU glycemic control: another can't miss quality measure bites the dust. 2009. Available at: http://www.leapfroggroup.org/media/file/Leapfrog-ICU_Physician_Staffing_Fact_Sheet.pdf.
33. Burack JH, Impellizzeri P, Homel P, et al. Public reporting of surgical mortality: a survey of New York State cardiothoracic surgeons. Ann Thorac Surg 1999;68(4):1195–200.
34. Jha AK, Orav EJ, Epstein AM. Low-quality, high-cost hospitals, mainly in South, care for sharply higher shares of elderly black, Hispanic, and medicaid patients. Health Aff (Millwood) 2011;30(10):1904–11.
35. Rosenthal MB, Frank RG, Li Z, et al. Early experience with pay-for-performance: from concept to practice. JAMA 2005;294(14):1788–93.
36. Lindenauer PK, Remus D, Roman S, et al. Public reporting and pay for performance in hospital quality improvement. N Engl J Med 2007;356(5):486–96.
37. Jha AK, Joynt KE, Orav EJ, et al. The long-term effect of premier pay for performance on patient outcomes. N Engl J Med 2012;366(17):1606–15.
38. Witter S, Fretheim A, Kessy FL, et al. Paying for performance to improve the delivery of health interventions in low- and middle-income countries. Cochrane Database Syst Rev 2012;(2):CD007899.
39. Mehrotra A, Damberg CL, Sorbero ME, et al. Pay for performance in the hospital setting: what is the state of the evidence? Am J Med Qual 2009;24(1):19–28.
40. National Healthcare Quality Report 2011. U.S. Department of Health and Human Services. Agency for Healthcare Research and Quality. Rockville (MD): AHRQ Publication No. 12-0005. March 2012. Available at: www.ahrq.gov/qual/qrdr11.htm.

41. Galvin R, Milstein A. Large employers' new strategies in health care. N Engl J Med 2002;347(12):939–42.
42. Parikh A, Huang SA, Murthy P, et al. Quality improvement and cost savings after implementation of the Leapfrog intensive care unit physician staffing standard at a community teaching hospital. Crit Care Med 2012;40(10):2754–9.
43. Pronovost PJ, Needham DM, Waters H, et al. Intensive care unit physician staffing: financial modeling of the Leapfrog standard. Crit Care Med 2004;32(6):1247–53.
44. The Leapfrog Group. ICU Physician Staffing (IPS). 2008.
45. Statement on ensuring correct patient, correct site, and correct procedure surgery. Bull Am Coll Surg 2002;87(12):26.
46. Wrong site surgery and the Universal Protocol. Bull Am Coll Surg 2006;91(11):63.
47. Stahel PF, Sabel AL, Victoroff MS, et al. Wrong-site and wrong-patient procedures in the universal protocol era: analysis of a prospective database of physician self-reported occurrences. Arch Surg 2010;145(10):978–84.
48. Vital signs: central line-associated blood stream infections—United States, 2001, 2008, and 2009. MMWR Morb Mortal Wkly Rep 2011;60(8):243–8.
49. Rau J. Hospitals treating the poor hardest hit by readmissions penalties. 2012. Available at: http://www.kaiserhealthnews.org/Stories/2012/August/13/hospitals-treating-poor-hardest-hit-readmissions-penalties.aspx.
50. Philbin EF, Dec GW, Jenkins PL, et al. Socioeconomic status as an independent risk factor for hospital readmission for heart failure. Am J Cardiol 2001;87(12):1367–71.
51. Joynt KE, Orav EJ, Jha AK. Thirty-day readmission rates for Medicare beneficiaries by race and site of care. JAMA 2011;305(7):675–81.
52. Van WC, Bennett C, Jennings A, et al. Proportion of hospital readmissions deemed avoidable: a systematic review. CMAJ 2011;183(7):E391–402.
53. Van WC, Jennings A, Taljaard M, et al. Incidence of potentially avoidable urgent readmissions and their relation to all-cause urgent readmissions. CMAJ 2011;183(14):E1067–72.
54. Kahn JM, Rubenfeld GD, Rohrbach J, et al. Cost savings attributable to reductions in intensive care unit length of stay for mechanically ventilated patients. Med Care 2008;46(12):1226–33.
55. Hall WB, Willis LE, Medvedev S, et al. The implications of long-term acute care hospital transfer practices for measures of in-hospital mortality and length of stay. Am J Respir Crit Care Med 2012;185(1):53–7.
56. Kahn JM, Benson NM, Appleby D, et al. Long-term acute care hospital utilization after critical illness. JAMA 2010;303(22):2253–9.

Enhancing the Quality of Care in the Intensive Care Unit

A Systems Engineering Approach

Steven P. Tropello, MD, MS[a], Alan D. Ravitz, MS, PE[b], Mark Romig, MD[c], Peter J. Pronovost, MD, PhD[a,c,d], Adam Sapirstein, MD[a,c,*]

KEYWORDS

- Systems engineering • Intensive care units • Health care quality
- Health care systems • Patient harms

KEY POINTS

- Health care systems must embrace a more formal process to deal with rising costs, complexity, and patient harms.
- Systems engineering methodologies have been applied successfully to solve other major industrial problems.
- The systems engineering process reproducibly formalizes defining system problems and goals and prioritizes development of a system to meet those goals.
- The Patient Care Program Acute Care Initiative project will use a holistic patient-centered systems engineering approach to reengineer the intensive care unit.
- Application of systems engineering principles to the Patient Care Program Acute Care Initiative project will help enhance the quality of care and reduce patient harms.

Funding sources: This work has been funded by The Gordon and Betty Moore Foundation and The Systems Institute of Johns Hopkins University. Additional support includes: Mr Ravitz: Agency for Healthcare Research and Quality Grant 1R18HS020460; Dr Romig: Department of Anesthesiology & Critical Care Medicine; Dr Pronovost: none; Dr Sapirstein: Department of Anesthesiology & Critical Care Medicine.
Conflict of interest: Dr Tropello, Mr Ravitz, Dr Romig, and Dr Sapirstein have no conflicts to report. Dr Pronovost has received funding from the Agency for Healthcare Research and Quality, the National Institutes of Health, RAND, and the Commonwealth Fund for research related to measuring and improving patient safety; honoraria from various hospitals and health care systems and the Leigh Bureau to speak on quality and safety; consultancy with the Association for Professionals in Infection Control and Epidemiology, and book royalties for *Safe Patients, Smart Hospitals: How One Doctor's Checklist Can Help Us Change Health Care From the Inside Out.*
[a] The Armstrong Institute for Patient Safety and Quality, Johns Hopkins University School of Medicine, 650 East Pratt Street, Baltimore, MD 21202, USA; [b] The Johns Hopkins University Applied Physics Laboratory, Johns Hopkins University, 11100 Johns Hopkins Road, Laurel, MD 20901, USA; [c] The Department of Anesthesiology & Critical Care Medicine, Johns Hopkins University School of Medicine, 1800 Orleans Street, Baltimore, MD 21287, USA; [d] The Department of Health Policy and Management, Johns Hopkins Bloomberg School of Public Health, Johns Hopkins University School of Nursing, Johns Hopkins Carey Business School, 615 North Wolfe Street, Baltimore, MD 21205, USA
* Corresponding author. 1800 Orleans Street, Zayed 9127, Baltimore, MD 21287.
E-mail address: asapirs1@jhmi.edu

Crit Care Clin 29 (2013) 113–124
http://dx.doi.org/10.1016/j.ccc.2012.10.009 **criticalcare.theclinics.com**

INTRODUCTION

Health care technologies in the United States have been growing rapidly over the last half century, leading to ever-increasing treatment options, costs, and complexity. When compared with other industries, such as aerospace, defense, and information technology, the health care industry has underused systems engineering (SE) to help facilitate the design and reengineering of its complex network of systems.[1,2] In SE, the designers and users of a system describe the desired goals and priorities, and then create a system to meet those goals. This is not the case in health care. Technology companies, rather than clinicians and patients, usually design technologies. It is often unclear what goal or problem the technology solves or if it improves care. Technologies are often not well integrated into the overall care system. Technologies fail to talk to each other and may consume valuable clinician time and add to health care costs. Without proven benefit, many health care technologies have the potential to make care less safe and increase the risks for patient harm.[3] We hypothesize that the application of SE can significantly improve patient safety.

Recently, the Centers for Medicare and Medicaid Services launched a national effort to reduce 9 types of patient harm. These harms include adverse drug events, catheter-associated urinary tract infections, central line-associated bloodstream infections, fall injuries, pressure ulcers, surgical site infections, venous thromboembolisms, ventilator-associated pneumonias, and obstetric adverse events.[4] This is only a limited list, because health care experts have identified several other patient harms. The health care industry is addressing these harms as if each one occurs in isolation or independently, when they are interdependent. For example, patients who do not receive early and frequent mobilization are at risk for both pressure ulcers and venous thromboembolism, and it is no surprise that patient harms cluster, because 1 harm leads to another. Yet nobody wants these harms to occur: not patients, not clinicians, not insurers, not technology companies. Still, the approach of health care to reduce harm relies on ever-increasing heroism of clinicians rather than designing safe systems. Current approaches at harm reduction often rely on brute force efforts and clinicians work on preventing 1 or 2 harms, although patients are at risk for many more harms. Without a systems approach to prevent these harms, improvement efforts are typically independent initiatives by providers and patients.[5,6]

The Armstrong Institute of Johns Hopkins University School of Medicine in conjunction with the Gordon and Betty Moore Foundation and the University of California San Francisco is beginning a 2-year initiative, called the Patient Care Program Acute Care Initiative (PCPACI). The goal of the PCPACI is to enhance the quality of care and reduce patient harms in the intensive care unit (ICU) by using a holistic transdisciplinary patient-centered SE approach to reengineer the ICU. The PCPACI plans to significantly improve measures of clinical processes and outcomes for ICU-acquired deep venous thrombosis-pulmonary embolism, delirium and weakness, ventilator-associated injuries, and central line-associated blood stream infections (CLABSI) by integrating clinical information systems, integrating clinical equipment, designing or reengineering interprofessional care team workflows, and incorporating patient-family goals.

The first part of this article provides a brief overview of SE methodology, focusing on the overarching SE core principles used within all SE methodologies and domains. In sharp contrast to health care, SE methods begin by defining goals and desired outcomes and develop forward. The second part of the article proposes the application of SE methodologies to the PCPACI, highlighting a few examples within the ICU-acquired weakness and early mobilization subsystems.

OVERVIEW OF SE METHODOLOGY

The origins of SE are not clear, but its core principles, or systems methodology, emerged to help manage the rapid growth of many complex systems. The International Council of Systems Engineering (INCOSE) describes the history of the field and offers this comprehensive definition of a system as

> *...a construct or collections of different elements that together produce results not obtainable by the elements alone. The elements, or parts, can include people, hardware, software, facilities, policies, and documents; that is, all things required to produce systems-level results. The results include system level qualities, properties, characteristics, functions, behavior and performance. The value added by the system as a whole, beyond that contributed independently by the parts, is primarily created by the relationship among the parts; that is, how they are interconnected.*[7,8]

At some level, SE principles have been used since antiquity to build complex systems such as the Egyptian pyramids and Roman cities and aqueducts. During World War II, various military systems became increasingly complex and difficult to manage without a formal methodology to evaluate the performance of the whole system, its subsystems, and the relationships among these components.[9] In this period, formal definitions and principles of SE were codified in textbooks and successfully applied to military and other systems.

The modern world is even more complex and the application of SE methodologies has grown and broadened into many domains such as computer information systems, spacecraft systems, financial systems, transportation systems, and many others.[9,10] We face a series of multidisciplinary challenges in designing an integrated system for the ICU. SE principles and best practices are focused on managing complex development efforts involving a diverse set of domains. For the PCPACI ICU project, the development team includes stakeholders from different domains, including clinical care, patients and families, human factors, computer engineering, information technology, health care economics, and epidemiology. The holistic approach to system development used by SEs ensures that expertise of each of these disciplines is factored into system design, capabilities, and life-cycle sustainment. Although each domain has developed a set of unique tools and methodologies, all use common core principles when developing a systems-based solution. All SE approaches to improving complex systems include the following phases[9,10]:

1. System concept development
2. Requirements analysis
3. Functional definition
4. Implementation
5. Verification and validation
6. Iteration

System Concept Development

The first phase in developing a new system is defining the problem(s), stakeholder(s), and goal(s). Although it may seem trivial, this first step is important, because it helps set scope and boundaries. A problem that is not clearly defined and concise can squander resources and lead to an ineffective and inefficient system solution. Conversely, if a problem is too narrowly defined, it can result in a system that lacks essential functions. Stakeholders are individuals or groups who may be directly or indirectly involved in any part of a system, and it is essential to identify all stakeholders early in the process so they can participate in defining system scope and other phases of system development. The completed system must achieve its desired goals. The goals must be clear, concise, and prioritized; the goals help define necessary and unnecessary system functions. Commonly, the goals also inform the metrics needed to validate an implemented system. For example, when developing a new ventilator system, a goal might be reduction of ventilator-associated injuries. Metrics used to validate such a ventilator system should include use of evidence-based therapies and rates of acute respiratory distress syndrome and ventilator-associated pneumonia.

Requirements Analysis

Requirements analysis is a phase in which stakeholders, informed by the problem statement and goals, state their requirements for a system: how the system will be used, where it will be used, who the users are, what is needed to support and maintain the system. Systems engineers distinguish necessary from desired features and begin to identify resource constraints. Engineers resolve conflicts between the requirements of different stakeholders. To achieve this goal, systems engineers engage stakeholders using a variety of methods, including individual interviews, focus groups, workshops, and surveys. Mandatory system requirements emerge from the problem statement and goals. Acceptable and appropriately functioning systems typically satisfy all the mandatory requirements. Furthering the example of a new ventilator system, an intensivist's requirement could be stated as "no patients should receive harmful tidal volumes." A resource constraint within this example would be that respiratory therapists are not available every minute of the day to identify patients receiving harmful tidal volumes. Commonly, stakeholder requirements conflict with resource constraints. These discrepancies are addressed in the functional definition phase of system development.

Functional Definition

The functional definition phase of system development defines what the system should do. During this phase, subsystems of the whole system are mapped out along with their individual and interdependent inputs, ideal functions, and expected outputs. Common tools used are block diagrams, flow diagrams, object-oriented models, computer simulations, and prototype designs of graphical user interfaces (GUIs) (ie, computer application displays). During this phase, systems engineers automate, standardize, and install redundancy within critical, complex, or time-consuming system functions. In the example of a new ventilator system, one of the functions might be for the processor subsystem to receive an input of patient height and automatically calculate ideal (ie. safe) tidal volume ranges, which would then be displayed on the user interface subsystem to inform the providers.

Implementation

In the implementation phase, the system is developed and built. Subsystems such as computer programs, processes to support human performance, and physical materials are built and tested. This subsystem testing is followed by integration into the overall system, which is then tested as a whole. At the end of this phase, the system should function and produce the expected outputs. Systems engineers begin collecting and monitoring predefined metrics in order to validate the overall function of the system.

Verification and Validation

One of the most important phases of system development is verification and validation throughout the life cycle of the system. Systems engineers use predefined metrics to verify that the completed system is fulfilling stated goal(s) and functioning in an optimal fashion. After verification, the validation process is conducted when users operate the system in a simulated or real environment and perform evaluations. Data often expose unanticipated system weaknesses or opportunities for improvement. Feedback from this process and any operational use is available for an iterative process in which systems engineers can evolve the system.

Iteration

Iteration ideally takes place in a parallel fashion throughout all phases of systems development and should not be limited to implemented systems. For example, stakeholders may change their requirements during the implementation phase of system development and engineers would iterate back through the functional definition phase with new requirements as they continue to work in parallel on system implementation. Changing or adding new requirements often requires compromises between stakeholders, because they can increase costs and development times of a project.

APPLICATION OF SE METHODOLOGY

The PCPACI set out to enhance the quality of care and reduce patient harms in the ICU by using SE methodology. The following sections provide examples of how the PCPACI has used and will continue to use SE methodology. For brevity and consistency, examples focus on ICU-acquired weakness and early mobilization subsystems.

System Concept Development

A simple problem statement is that ICUs often deliver poor quality of care, which causes harm to and disrespects patients and negatively affects their family members. The PCPACI has initially limited the problem scope and set goals to focus clinical improvements in ICU-acquired deep venous thrombosis-pulmonary embolism, ICU-acquired delirium, ICU-acquired weakness, ventilator-associated injuries, CLABSI, and disrespectful and undignified care. **Fig. 1** shows the system scope and highlights how, in the long-term, the PCPACI will work to iteratively scale the system to prevent other ICU-related harms and implement the system across ICUs in many health care systems. The initial system developed in the PCPACI will be validated in the surgical ICU (SICU) at The Johns Hopkins Hospital over a 2-year period ending in 2014. The project includes long-term goals to implement and validate the system in other ICU subspecialty environments such as cardiac, medical, and neurologic ICUs. The project has a goal to implement the system within other academic and community hospital systems.

The PCPACI has placed stakeholder involvement at the core of its system, with an emphasis on the goals of patients and their families. **Fig. 2** shows some of the stakeholders involved in the PCPACI and shows how the patient and their family members are the most important stakeholders when considering system development.

The PCPACI has several goals for the system. Most of the goals are specific to particular harms, such as ICU-acquired weakness and early mobilization subsystems. Three examples of specific goals are:

1. The system will permit patients and family members to participate in patient care to the degree at which it would not interfere or negatively affect care
2. The system will provide early and appropriate physical rehabilitation activities to at least 70% of all patients in the ICU
3. The system will improve physical function, compared with best prehospital or inpatient physical performance, in at least 20% of all patients in the ICU

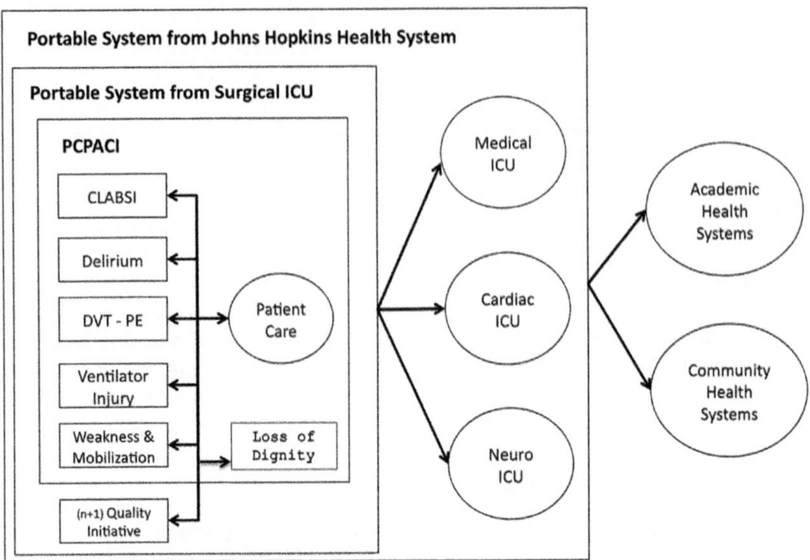

Fig. 1. Initial scope and future scalability of the PCPACI system. The diagram shows the 5 clinical patient care elements as well as loss of dignity that are initially targeted in the surgical ICU. In future phases, additional care elements will be added incrementally as shown by the (n + 1) quality initiative and the system will be implemented in other ICU environments on campus. The system will be implemented in other academic health systems (University of San Francisco) and community health systems.

The first goal is pertinent to the entire system, whereas the second and third goals are specific to the ICU-acquired weakness and early mobilization subsystems. The second and third goals exemplify how clear goal definition during this phase of system development helps to create performance metrics, such as percentage of patients able to participate in physical rehabilitation, which systems engineers use during the system validation phase.

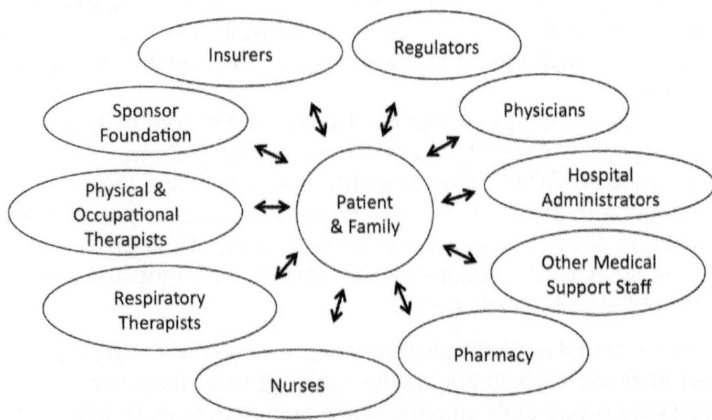

Fig. 2. PCPACI stakeholders. The figure places the patient and family in the center of a group of stakeholders in the PCPACI system. Other major stakeholders in the system are shown around the patient and family.

Requirements Analysis

The requirements analysis phase of the PCPACI system is an ongoing process as stakeholders individually, or in groups, continue to further refine system requirements or conceive of additional requirements. Systems engineers do not include every requirement in the functional definitions, because, although it may be important to a specific stakeholder, a requirement may not help to achieve any stated system goal(s). For example, a PCPACI stakeholder required real-time calorimetry on all ventilated patients. Although real-time calorimetry likely has some usefulness, it would not help fulfill any system goal(s).

The PCPACI development group has provided 1 mandatory and complex system requirement in which patients and their family members must be able to express their desired level of patient care participation in real time and the system should adapt to their desired level of participation. For example, a patient's partner may want to participate in passive range-of-motion physical therapy for a given day. Three examples of related requirements are:

1. Family members who would like to participate in physical therapy must first complete an appropriately designed training course
2. Patients and family members may participate in patient care activities, but their participation must not interfere with patient care as determined by care providers
3. Nurses may initiate physical therapy using activity plans prescribed by consulting physical therapists if they meet inclusion criteria and are not excluded by their physical condition (**Box 1**).

System requirements for clinical interventions are provided by many stakeholders, including physicians, nurses, physical therapists, and administrators, and are guided by patient safety and regulatory considerations. For example, all stakeholders believed that the most responsible path for involving family members in physical therapy activities was to require a minimum level of basic physical therapy training via frequent courses or online training modules.

Box 1
Example of exclusion criteria for early physical rehabilitation protocol

1. Richmond Agitation and Sedation Scale = –4, –5, or 3 or greater
2. Poor oxygenation: pulse oximetry less than 88%, F_{IO_2} (fraction of inspired oxygen) greater than 60%, positive end-expiratory pressure greater than 10 cm H_2O or high frequency oscillation ventilation
3. Tachypnea: respiratory rate greater than 45 breaths per minute
4. Acidosis: recent arterial pH less than 7.25
5. Hypotension: mean arterial pressure (MAP) less than 55 mm Hg, increase in vasopressor dose within the past 2 hours, norepinephrine greater than 0.15 μg/kg/min, dopamine greater than 15 μg/kg/min, phenylephrine greater than 1 μg/kg/min, vasopressin greater than 0.02 units/min
6. Hypertension: MAP greater than 140 mm Hg, any dose of a continuous intravenous infusion of nitroglycerin, nitroprusside, nicardipine, diltiazem, esmolol, or labetolol
7. New deep vein thrombosis: duration of anticoagulation less than 36 hours (only applicable for rehabilitation to affected limb and for ambulation)

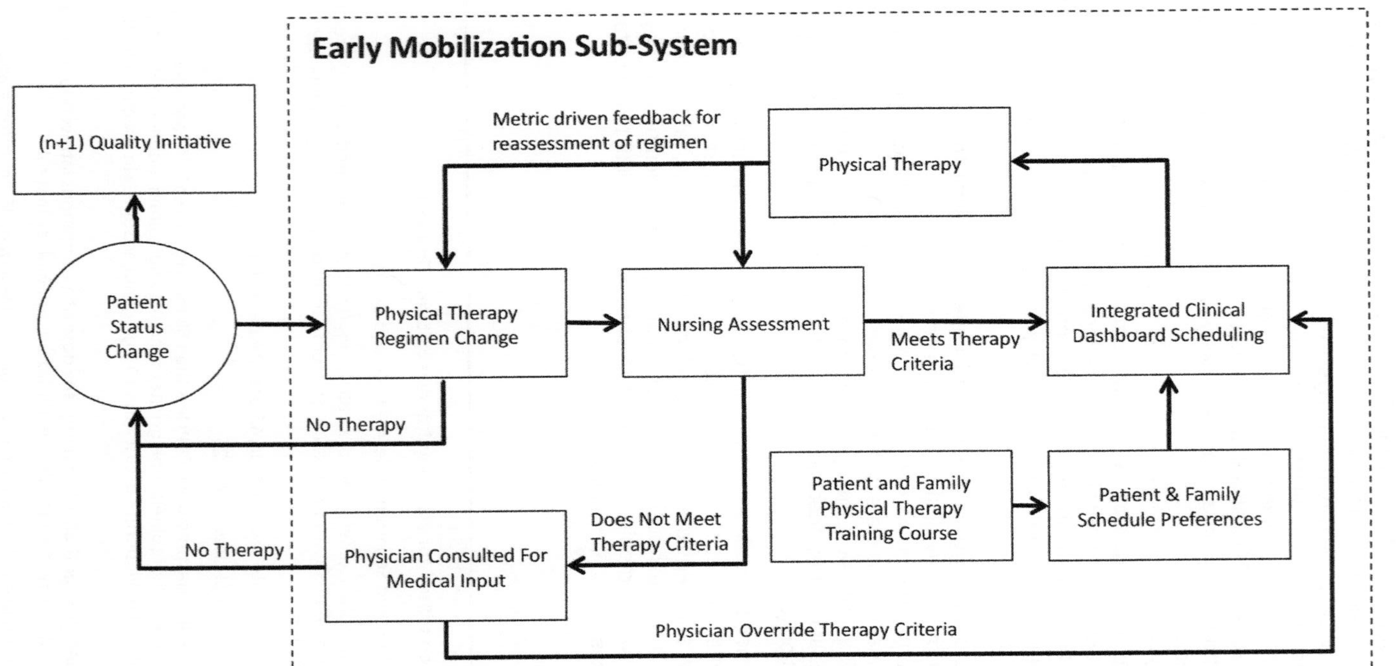

Fig. 3. Early mobilization subsystem functional block. The figure presents sequential steps in the systems approach to performing early mobilization of patients in the ICU. Patients must meet criteria for the therapy and the system considers patient and family preferences and participation. Information regarding scheduling and performance of mobilization is displayed on the ICDS, and metrics are collected for ongoing reassessment of the therapy. If the status of the patient changes, this is considered in the therapeutic evaluation. The process can be expanded to other (n + 1) quality initiatives.

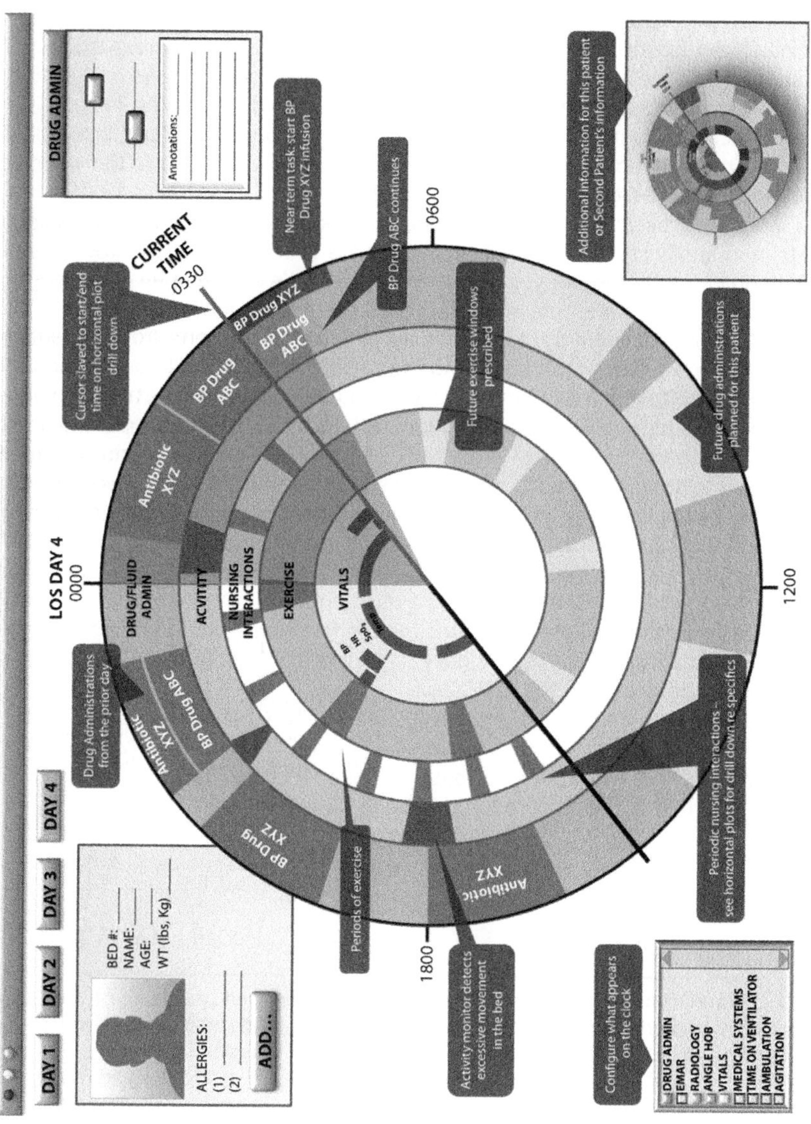
DAY 1
DAY 2
DAY 3
DAY 4
BED #:
NAME:
AGE:
WT (lbs, Kg)
ALLERGIES:
(1)
(2)
ADD...
DRUG ADMIN
Annotations:
LOS DAY 4
0000
0600
1200
1800
CURRENT TIME
0330
DRUG/FLUID ADMIN
ACVITITY
NURSING INTERACTIONS
EXERCISE
VITALS
BP
HR
SpO2
RR
Antibiotic XYZ
BP Drug ABC
BP Drug XYZ
Drug Administrations from the prior day
Cursor slaved to start/end time on horizontal plot drill down
Near term task: start BP Drug XYZ infusion
BP Drug ABC continues
Future exercise windows prescribed
Future drug administrations planned for this patient
Additional information for this patient or Second Patient's information
Periodic nursing interactions - see horizontal plots for drill down re specifics
Periods of exercise
Activity monitor detects excessive movement in the bed
Configure what appears on the clock
DRUG ADMIN
EMAR
RADIOLOGY
ANGLE HOB
VITALS
MEDICAL SYSTEMS
TIME ON VENTILATOR
AMBULATION
AGITATION

Functional Definition

The functional definition phase of the PCPACI system is planned to continue through 2012. Stakeholders and systems engineers are applying stakeholder requirements to formulate a detailed model of a functional system. Engineering resources and expertise comes from the Johns Hopkins University Applied Physics Laboratory (APL) and Whiting School of Engineering, and performance measurement expertise comes from the Bloomberg School of Public Health. APL has collaborated with Johns Hopkins Medicine (JHM) for several decades and APL engineers and JHM researchers and clinicians have successfully built a wide range of successful devices and systems. Engineers and computer scientists are working to clearly define the integration of necessary clinical information systems with clinical equipment and configure clinical processes and work flow. **Fig. 3** shows a functional block diagram of the work flow and scheduling for the early mobilization subsystem.

The integrated clinical dashboard system (ICDS) included in **Fig. 3** facilitates patients' and family members' ability to coordinate with nurses on desired times for participation in physical therapy. For example, a patient's partner may prefer physical therapy to take place during the afternoon because they would be able to leave work during their lunch break. Within reason, the nurse can facilitate scheduling this request for participation in physical therapy using the ICDS.

Patients in the ICU are at risk for many harms, but clinicians have not clearly defined all of them or the strategies to prevent them. However, some harms and prevention strategies have been described. The ICDS will provide visual alignment of specific tasks needed to prevent defined patient harms with the relevant data regarding those harms. For example, early rehabilitation may affect venous thromboembolism, ventilator-related injuries, and acquired weakness. A significant investment is planned to build the ICDS, which will serve as an interface to display, analyze, and inform stakeholders of all PCPACI subsystems. Patients and family members will receive an e-tablet device that will provide access to the family-specific portion of the ICDS and facilitate data input and display daily therapies and interventions. **Fig. 4** shows an early prototype design of the ICDS GUI.

The ICDS GUI includes several clockfaces to visually enhance time-sensitive functions within different subsystems. It is the goal of the ICDS to efficiently display functions that will improve performance in subsystems in which evidence-based practices can prevent harm to patients. In addition, the ICDS will integrate data and communications generated by the patient and family members, such as facilitating scheduling physical therapy with nurses. The right side of **Fig. 4** shows the period available for future exercise during which nurses would be available for physical therapy and

Fig. 4. Integrated clinical dashboard GUI prototype. An idealized prototype of the GUI for ICU confusion awareness and management is shown. The ICDS analyzes patient data and presents information in a 24-hour-clock format. The format uses a series of concentric circles for each domain, with vital signs at the core and radiating outward to drug administration. The display features a current time line (*red line*), which sweeps in a clockwise fashion. The GUI shows information related to each domain over the previous 12 hours and uses color coding to indicate expected performance or results (*green*) or issues of concern (*red*) such as excessive patient activity. Pending tasks or events that will occur over the next 12 hours are displayed in advance of the current time indicator. More detailed information about events can be obtained by selecting a field. The icon in the bottom right corner allows users to select other displays that specifically address information related to prevention of other patient harms.

patients or family members could schedule times to have physical therapy. This facility would allow better coordination of family participation with patient care.

Implementation

The implementation phase of the PCPACI system is planned to continue until April, 2013. Engineers at the APL have started programming some parts of the ICDS and are working to integrate the ICDS with current clinical information systems at the Johns Hopkins University Health System. The PCPACI plans to implement an early prototype system by May, 2013 and to begin collecting metrics after that time for system validation.

Verification and Validation

The PCPACI will begin collecting standardized data in the SICU at Johns Hopkins Hospital in November, 2012. These data will establish a performance and incidence baseline that will enable comparison to determine if the new PCPACI system is improving the quality of patient care. Examples of benchmark metrics related to ICU-acquired weakness and early mobilization include incidence rates of ICU-acquired weakness, percentage of patients receiving early physical rehabilitation activities, and percentage of patients with improved physical mobility compared with their best prehospital and inpatient physical performances. Teams of researchers will collect these data throughout the project period. This process will allow comparison of data quality from automated electronic sources with manually abstracted data. As time passes, the PCPACI will strive to improve metric performance data relative to the new system and not the previous SICU system. This push for further performance improvement will take place through incremental system evolution as data highlight system weaknesses or strengths. Systems engineers will work in an iterative stepwise fashion, using all phases of SE methodology, to enhance the system and maximize performance throughout the life cycle of the system.

SUMMARY

Our rapidly expanding and fragmented health care systems are unsustainable. Our health care system too often harms patients, is too costly, and too often relies on the heroism of clinicians rather than good system design. Recent analyses from the Institute of Medicine suggest that about one-third of health care spending, or $750 billion, is wasted on inefficiencies and does nothing to make patients better.[3] New financial pressures and government policies will force changes in the health care industry to improve on inefficiencies, poor quality, and negative patient outcomes. If we (the stakeholders and advocates for patient care quality) do not actively collaborate to design improvements in performance and delivery of health care, then changes will be driven not by careful design and testing but rather by financial constraints.

We believe that the reengineering of our health care systems requires an SE approach using SE methodologies that have been developed and have proved successful in a myriad of other industries over the last half century.[1,9] We have highlighted the core principles of all SE methodologies and how these principles facilitate a more holistic and comprehensive system design and life-cycle development. We have further shown our current application of these principles to the PCPACI system, with the goal of enhancing the quality of care and reducing patient harms in the ICU. By using a holistic and comprehensive systems approach to improving quality and reducing patient harms in the ICU, the PCPACI will develop a system that does not address harms via fragmented solutions but a system that is capable of addressing all harms and adapting functions to address future patient and family goals. We hope that stakeholders of other health care systems can use this systems approach to take action and reengineer their own systems.

REFERENCES

1. Pronovost PJ, Bo-Linn GW. Preventing patient harms through systems of care. JAMA 2012;308(8):769–70.
2. Mathews SC, Pronovost PJ. The need for systems integration in health care. JAMA 2011;305(9):934–5.
3. Institute of Medicine. Best care at lower cost: the path to continuously learning health care in America. Washington, DC: The National Academies Press; 2012.
4. Health and human services, partnership for patients: making care safer. 2012. Available at: http://www.healthcare.gov/compare/partnership-for-patients/safety/index.html. Accessed September 27, 2012.
5. Pronovost PJ, Goeschel CA, Colantuoni E, et al. Sustaining reductions in catheter related bloodstream infections in Michigan intensive care units: observational study. BMJ 2010;340:c309.
6. Vasilevskis EE, Ely EW, Speroff T, et al. Reducing iatrogenic risks: ICU-acquired delirium and weakness–crossing the quality chasm. Chest 2010;138(5):1224–33.
7. INCOSE, A brief history of systems engineering. 2012. Available at: http://www.incose.org/mediarelations/briefhistory.aspx. Accessed September 27, 2012.
8. INCOSE, A consensus of the INCOSE fellows. 2012. Available at: http://www.incose.org/practice/fellowsconsensus.aspx. Accessed September 27, 2012.
9. Kossiakoff A, Sweet WN, Seymour S, et al. Systems engineering: principles and practice. Hoboken, NJ: John Wiley; 2011.
10. Gibson JE, Scherer WT, Gibson WF. How to do systems analysis. Hoboken, NJ: Wiley-Interscience; 2007.

Index

Note: Page numbers of article titles are in **boldface** type.

B

Bloodstream infections (BSIs)
  described, 1
BSIs. *See* Bloodstream infections (BSIs)

C

Catheter-associated urinary tract infections (CAUTIs)
  in ICU, **19–32**
    epidemiology of, 20–22
    financial implications of, 20
    microbial causes of, 21
    mortality related to, 20
    pathogenesis of, 20
    prevalence of, 19
    prevention of, 23–27
      alternatives to indwelling urinary catheters in, 26
      aseptic techniques for insertion and maintenance of urinary catheters in, 26–27
      bundles and collaboratives in, 27
      general strategies in, 23–24
      limitation of use of urinary catheters in, 24–26
      perioperative management of urinary catheters in, 26
      use of anti-infective catheters in, 27
    risk factors for, 21–22
    surveillance for, 22–23
CAUTIs. *See* Catheter-associated urinary tract infections (CAUTIs)
Centers for Medicare and Medicaid Services (CMS), 94–95, 100–101, 104–106
  VBP and, 94–95, 101
Central line–associated bloodstream infection (CLABSI)
  zero
    in ICU, **1–9**
      described, 1–7
CLABSI. *See* Central line–associated bloodstream infection (CLABSI)
Clostridium difficile
  described, 11–12
Clostridium difficile infection
  in ICU, **11–18**
    epidemiology of, 12–13
    outcomes related to, 13–14
    prevention of
      antimicrobial use restrictions in, 15–16
      environmental cleaning and disinfection in, 15

Crit Care Clin 29 (2013) 125–128
http://dx.doi.org/10.1016/S0749-0704(12)00095-4 criticalcare.theclinics.com
0749-0704/13/$ – see front matter

Clostridium (*continued*)
measures for health care workers, patients, and visitors in, 14–15
probiotics use in, 16
CMS. *See* Centers for Medicare and Medicaid Services (CMS)
Collaborative intensive care unit (ICU) networks
described, 77–78
essential elements of, 79–85
examples of, 78–79
in quality of care improvement, **77–89**
benefits of, 75
future research related to, 85–86
unintended consequences of, 75

D

Delirium
in ICU, **51–65**
described, 51–52
prevention of, 55–61
ABCDE approach to, 59–61
early mobilization of patient in, 57–58
pain management in, 57
pharmacologic interventions in, 58–59
sedative management in, 55–57
sleep improvements in, 58
risk factors for, 52–53
in non-ICU patients
prevention of, 53–55

H

HAIs. *See* Health care–associated infections (HAIs)
Health care–associated infections (HAIs)
described, 1

I

Intensive care unit (ICU)
C. difficile infection in, **11–18**. *See also Clostridium difficile* infection, in ICU
CAUTIs in, **19–32**. *See also* Catheter-associated urinary tract infections (CAUTIs), in ICU
collaborative networks in
in quality of care improvement, **77–89**. *See also* Collaborative intensive care unit (ICU) networks
delirium in, **51–65**. *See also* Delirium, in ICU
quality of care in
enhancing, **113–124**. *See also* Systems engineering (SE), in enhancing quality of care in ICU
sedation and mobility in, **67–75**
VACs in, **33–50**. *See also* Ventilator-associated complications (VACs), in ICU
VAP in, **33–50**. *See also* Ventilator-associated pneumonia (VAP), in ICU

VBP effects on quality of life of patients in, **91–112**. *See* Centers for Medicare and Medicaid Services (CMS); Value-based purchasing (VBP)
zero CLABSI in, **1–9**

M

Mobility
sedation and
in ICU, **67–75**

N

National Quality Forum (NQF)
performance measures and, 92–99
in VBP, **91–112**. *See also* Centers for Medicare and Medicaid Services (CMS); Value-based purchasing (VBP)
NQF. *See* National Quality Forum (NQF)

P

Performance measures
effects on quality of life and patient outcomes in ICU
mechanisms of, 95, 100, 104–106
NQF and, 92–99

Q

Quality of care
in ICU
collaborative networks in improving, **77–89**. *See also* Collaborative intensive care unit (ICU) networks
enhancing, **113–124**. *See also* Systems engineering (SE), in enhancing quality of care in ICU

S

SE. *See* Systems engineering (SE)
Sedation
mobility and
in ICU, **67–75**
Systems engineering (SE)
in enhancing quality of care in ICU, **113–124**
described, 114
methodology of
application of, 117–123
functional definition in, 116, 122–123
implementation in, 116, 123
iteration in, 117
overview of, 115–117
requirements analysis in, 116, 119–121

Systems (*continued*)
system concept development in, 115–119
verification and validation in, 116–117, 123

U

Urinary tract infections (UTIs)
catheter-associated
in ICU, **19–32**. *See also* Catheter-associated urinary tract infections (CAUTIs), in ICU
in ICU
prevalence of, 19

V

VACs. *See* Ventilator-associated complications (VACs)
Value-based purchasing (VBP)
CMS and, 94–95, 101
in enhancing quality of care and patient outcomes in ICU, **91–112**
described, 91–92
evidence of, 106–108
future of, 108–109
measures of, 102–104
VAP. *See* Ventilator-associated pneumonia (VAP)
VBP. *See* Value-based purchasing (VBP)
Ventilator-associated complications (VACs)
in ICU, **33–50**. *See also* Ventilator-associated pneumonia (VAP), in ICU
prevention of
approaches to, 43–44
Ventilator-associated pneumonia (VAP)
in ICU, **33–50**
described, 33–35
prevention of
approaches to, 43–44
bundles in, 37–41
process elements in, 41–42
problematic definition of, 35–37

Printed and bound by CPI Group (UK) Ltd, Croydon, CR0 4YY

08/06/2025

01896873-0009